MW00511269

The Science of Destroying Adult ADHD

Stop Guessing, Quit Unnatural Treatments, and Attain Superhuman Focus

Michelle Martin

Table of Contents

Introduction

So you finally came to accept the fact that you have a medical condition known as ADHD. It took you a while to process what this diagnosis would mean for you, your performance at school or at work, and your interactions with other people going forward. Nevertheless, accepting that you had ADHD would give you access to treatments, therapy, and a community that would make this new journey worthwhile. However, while you may have accepted that you have ADHD, society has been less than kind. Not only do people question who you are (as if your personality was somehow affected), but they also question whether you have a serious condition or you are just making up a series of excuses.

With all of the medical research done studying this condition, there is still a society at large whose skepticism and ignorance about ADHD has translated to stigmatizing those who suffer from it. Let's face it—ADHD has become a taboo from which many seek to hide or distance themselves. This negative standpoint on the condition is due to the many myths about it that dominate social discourse. Perhaps we should take this time to bust a few of these myths, shall we?

Myth 1: ADHD isn't a real medical condition.

The fact is that ADHD is an actual medical condition recognized by the National Institutes of Health, the American Psychiatric Association, and the Centers for Disease Control and Prevention. In fact, since millions of children in the United States have been diagnosed with ADHD, it is seen to be one of the most common childhood conditions. Research has also shown that it is hereditary; a study showed that one out of four people with ADHD has a parent with the same condition (Morin, n.d.).

Therefore, since this is a real condition, we can finally quit questioning the legitimacy of a person's diagnosis and offer our support instead.

Myth 2: People with ADHD aren't pushing themselves hard enough.

There is a common misconception that individuals with ADHD are either lazy or aren't highly motivated to perform. The truth is that adults with ADHD are trying as hard as they can to pay attention. When we tell a person with ADHD to "just focus", it is the same as telling a right-handed person to start writing with their left hand; this would be extremely difficult. The inability to focus attentively for long periods of time is not an attitude issue. Instead, it has a lot to do with how differently a person with ADHD's brain is structured and how it functions.

Myth 3: People who have ADHD will never be able to focus.

While those with ADHD have difficulties focusing, they are still able to hyperfocus, especially when they are concentrating on something particularly interesting. In other words, it may be difficult for someone with ADHD to maintain concentration when dealing with mundane tasks. However, there may be some tasks that they completely absorb themselves in, thus helping them maintain focus a lot easier.

This book has been written to challenge some of these misconceptions surrounding ADHD and the experiences of those who have it. The aim is to prove that like with many other medical conditions, it is still possible to live a long and fulfilling life with ADHD.

The key to unlocking this life is changing your perspective about ADHD and the implications that are commonly associated with the condition. Instead of perceiving the condition as a problem that could set you back, why not view it as a gift that grants you the opportunity to strengthen specific skill sets, talents, passions, and knowledge? Even though you cannot focus your mind on all things, you have an extraordinary ability to hone in on certain aspects of life, work, school, and leisure activities that improve your level of creativity, emotional intelligence, interpersonal intuition, and leadership abilities.

Harnessing Your Superpower for Good

By simply recognizing that you are gifted, you can change your life in a meaningful way. For instance, understanding where your attention tends to lie can give you an indication of the topics, ideas, and activities that you are interested in or that you are extremely good at. Recognizing this gift will also create a shift in your mind, body, and soul as you expand your consciousness about who you are.

Many times, when those who have ADHD come to view their condition as a superpower, their entire self-perception changes. The mental blocks and negative self-talk that reminded them of their shortcomings suddenly disappears and is replaced with a subtle confidence and unshakable willpower to live free from the labels that are thrust upon them. Another incredible work of healing happens in their bodies. They discover that just like any other muscle, the brain can be trained to create new neural pathways and accept new information that it is fed on a continuous basis. Training the brain muscle (along with physical exercise) can significantly boost one's mental health, overall well-being, and self-esteem.

Lastly, when those with ADHD recognize their superpower, a miraculous change happens on a soul or emotional level. When you finally decide that nothing is wrong with you and that your diagnosis does not define who you are, the fear of being an outcast or struggling to progress in your life will vanish. Fear is only as real as we imagine it to be. This means that the more life and depth we give to our fears, the more they will morph into our reality.

The root of fear is never in something real—fear is always rooted in an illusion. The illusions of failing, being rejected, or not living to your full potential are not realistic predictions of your future or who you will become. Harnessing your superpower and changing your perspective on your condition will eradicate fear permanently.

At this point, you may be wondering what makes me qualified to speak on this subject or dare to change your mind on ADHD. I'm a relationship counselor who lives and works in Washington DC. Over the years, my career has given me an opportunity to acquaint myself with a wide spectrum of human emotions. Often, when I've reflected on my own life, I have found that many of the negative emotional blocks I've had stemmed from personal insecurities and past baggage. Finding patterns in my own behaviors had me curious about how other people process the full spectrum of emotion, from happiness to anger.

I started conducting my own study on relationship anxiety, pathological jealousy, the fear of abandonment, and unhealthy attachments. The results of the study are presented in my first book, *Anxiety in Relationships*. I had based the information on the real-life scenarios I faced in my work, my academic background, and extensive research on psychological factors contributing to relationship demise.

Apart from being a counselor who is passionately committed to the well-being of my patients, I am also a loving wife and a mom of three spectacularly bright kids. If my years of conducting research and writing books have taught me anything, it is that we as human beings are powerful enough to pick ourselves up from undesirable circumstances and take positive steps forward. Every one of us has the relentless spirit to conquer the odds that are stacked against us.

It is my intention in this book to show those who have ADHD (and the community of support around them) how to overcome undesirable circumstances by simply tapping into their inner strength. I will endeavor to show you how to dispel your mental and emotional blocks, rid of societal stigmas, eradicate personal fears, and avoid negative self-talk in order to live to your highest potential and fulfill your deepest desires!

Chapter 1:

I Am NOT My Diagnosis

It is time we break the silence about the stigma that comes when you live with ADHD. Stigma flourishes when we keep it hidden; however, as soon as we expose these misconceptions and stereotypes, they vanish into thin air, having no real substance to hold onto. The good news is that many people are starting to speak up, and gradually, the stigma surrounding ADHD is shrinking. There are, however, many myths that need to be denounced that bear no truth whatsoever.

According to psychotherapist Terry Matlen, who has written several books on this medical condition, many people still consider ADHD to be a personality trait or flaw in someone's character. Surprisingly, even those who have ADHD find it difficult to construct their identity outside of their diagnosis. In other words, we have two messages constantly flying back and forth between those who have the condition and the society around them. The one with ADHD says, "Who am I apart from my diagnosis?", and society at large says, "You are your diagnosis." Instead of seeing the medical condition as a part of a whole human being, there is a tendency for many people to live within the shadows of their medical condition due to their own decision to do so or after being pressured by others.

During the first few months or years after receiving the diagnosis, it is normal to go into shock and become consumed with many questions about who you are and who you will be in time. Suddenly, you think of the sacrifices you will have to make, the lifestyle adjustments approaching in the near future, and what you will and will not be allowed to do going forward. It's almost like preparing yourself for a storm that's about to close in on you and making sure that you are ready to settle for whatever may come. The preparation, strict routines, and lifestyle adjustments do more to change your personality than the diagnosis ever would.

Think about it for a second: You received a medical document saying you have ADHD, and then what series of events followed after that moment? Did your brain suddenly cave in on you worse than it did before you received this medical document? Or did you take it upon yourself to draft a new plan of action for your life that may have caused you to become someone else?

It is common for many adults who have either just received their diagnosis or haven't yet come to terms with it to change. How many of us actually question the need for this change? Why do you need to cut back on your social life? Why can't you continue working on that project or planning on progressing in that career? Who you are is not tied to what you have or don't have. Who you will be is also not tied to anything secondary in your life. Whether you have money or not or drive a fancy car, whether you are single or in a relationship, happy or sad, your identity is unscathed by what comes in and out of your life. Your diagnosis? That is not who you are. It is merely what you have, and since it is secondary, you are able to continue striving for purpose without it impeding your progress. Now, I know some of you are saying, "Michelle, it's easier said than done." But allow me to tell you this: Since your identity is more than the things around you, you are able to control the noise in your environment.

This is liberating. It means that you are not subjected to anything that doesn't align with who you are. For instance, you are not subjected to other people's ignorance about your condition. They may say you are lazy, but you know very well that being lazy is not a part of who you are. Now take this truth and apply it to other areas of your life where you find stigmatization. What about your work life? What are some of the stereotypes or criticisms you receive at work about your performance, productivity, or future prospects? Are these stereotypes and criticisms a fair critique of who you are? Do they align with your career goals? Do they magnify your passion for what you do? If the answer is no to all of these questions, then you can safely count the criticism as invalid and lacking real substance. You are not your diagnosis—you are so much more!

Focusing on the Wrong Thing

Reflect for a minute about some of the doubts or worries you have concerning your condition. If you would like to, you can write these doubts or worries down on a piece of paper as they pop up in your mind. Considering what came up, how many of these doubts or worries were other-centered, and how many of them were you-centered? Other-centered doubts or worries would sound something like this:

- "What if my boss doesn't consider me for a promotion?"

- "What if I am unable to help or support people?"
- "What if my future romantic partner disapproves of me?"
- "What if I am criticized in personal interactions?"
- "What if I can never relate to those closest to me?"

All of these what-ifs are focused on how you are or will be received by others, how others think of you, and whether or not you will ever be like others. It is possible to unknowingly center your diagnosis around others and neglect to see where you fit in or how you can empower yourself. Disapproval, failure, and rejection hurt. However, how much more painful is it to live in a body you have disapproved of or rejected?

By focusing on what you are constantly portraying to others, you spend less time focusing on what truly matters: what you think about yourself. It is natural to slowly morph into a people-pleaser when your attention is focused on how others perceive you. In your bid to preserve your self-image, you spend your effort making sure that your colleagues, friends, and family members approve of you. This also means that you are more likely to jump at the opportunity to show up for others than you would for yourself. Soon enough, you become a chameleon who is an expert at being anyone but themselves.

The most important thing you can do in life is decide that there is nothing wrong with you. A quick Google search on the definition of the word "wrong" will show you that it is impossible for anything to be wrong with you. Something or someone that is wrong is not living or operating in accordance with what is morally right or good. Something or someone that is wrong deviates from the truth or fact and is incorrect in their judgments or in how they choose to live their lives.

Living with ADHD doesn't make you defiant or defective in any way or form. Even ADHD as a medical condition isn't wrong. The condition simply describes how your brain functions and the implications of this unique rewiring. What could possibly be wrong with that? Most of the time, those living with ADHD spend time and energy focusing on correcting what they believe or feel is wrong about themselves.

While there is nothing particularly unseemly about seeking to improve yourself, it is, however, concerning when the reason why you seek self-improvement is due to an other-centered reality. In other words, if your life has become a game of proving that there's nothing wrong with you, you have entered a spiral of people-pleasing and people-seeking.

It should be enough for you to believe that there cannot possibly be anything wrong with you without seeking others to validate this belief. Remember who you are. Do you genuinely believe that there is something wrong with you? When you are busy with something that you deeply care about and unknowingly block out everything else, do you believe this is wrong?

While you cannot focus your mind on everything all of the time, there is an authenticity to how you prioritize what is important and deserving of your attention and what isn't. You choose to focus on the most exhilarating ideas, the most interesting facts, and the most engaging activities. Once again I ask, what could possibly be wrong with you?

Changing My Inner Script About My ADHD

When separating who you are from your diagnosis, it is also necessary to push the reset button on what you have told yourself about your own life. It is easy to forget this step because it doesn't really affect anything tangible. However, the self-talk that happens in your mind does affect your beliefs, values, and ideas about who you are and what you can or can't do. For instance, if you have spent a large part of your life believing that your diagnosis puts you at a disadvantage in some way, you may have created self-imposed limitations that have stopped you from aiming higher.

You may not know it, but you are significantly influenced by what you say to yourself. If you are prone to dismissing your own needs, chances are high that you are feeling unfulfilled or unheard in your life. On a surface level, you might think that this feeling of being unfulfilled stems from your frustration at work or the stress of everyday life, but in fact, the real reason is that you have silenced your own voice, needs, hopes, and goals.

All human beings have a natural desire to express themselves. Self-expression gives you the ability to distinguish yourself from other people, clearly articulate your personal needs and beliefs, and validate your unique ideas and philosophies on life. Being able to confidently express who you are should be your natural or default state and the beginning of a life filled with meaningful pursuits.

Sometimes, when societal pressures weigh you down or challenge your identity, you need to fight to maintain your convictions about who you are and speak up for yourself. One of the main mediums of expressing yourself is through speech. Using the spoken word, you have the ability to express the inner feelings, thoughts, and beliefs that make up your identity. How else are others supposed to know who you are if you don't communicate your unique attributes to them? But wait, here's an even bigger question: How are you able to express who you are when your own inner self-talk is negative?

Negative self-talk compromises your ability to express your identity. Most of the time, those who use negative self-talk project their fears, anxieties, and doubts onto others. For example, if you spend your time thinking about how disappointing you are, you are more likely to express a down-trodden or low-esteemed persona. Even though you know that you are not this down-trodden individual, the negative words that you repeat to yourself are influential enough to create negative behavioral patterns.

It's the same in the case of a person who appears shy or closed-off in public but when alone, is bursting with personality and energy. What they tell themselves about socializing or interacting with other people causes them to adopt withdrawn behaviors in public. Therefore, using negative self-talk (informed by a negative self-perception) can lead to you behaving and expressing yourself in ways that are not aligned with who you truly are and how you wish others to see you.

The Script: A Lens Through Which You Experience Your Life

Everyone, regardless of age, race, gender, religion, or political affiliation, has one thing in common: a life script. A life script is the story you hold about your life that has become the lens through which you perceive your reality. In other words, the way you are currently living, your lifestyle, and your daily activities are informed by this script or story. This script is also why some patterns or experiences continue to repeat themselves in your life.

The moment you found out that you had ADHD, you subconsciously began writing a script about what having ADHD would mean for you. As time went by, you continued to edit the script, adding new information about how you see the world post-diagnosis. Now, you are living a particular kind of lifestyle due to the script that you have been forming in your mind. What you love about your life, your work, and your interactions with others is all written in this script. However, what you dislike, fear, or are ashamed of about your life, work, and interactions with others are also recorded.

Therefore, coming to terms with who you are and your life with ADHD requires you to reflect on your script. The most influential way for you to experience something new in your life is to actually incorporate this new experience as part of your script. Fortunately, your script can always be rewritten to include what you want to see instead of what you fear or dread. Ideally, we all want a life where we are totally fulfilled and all of our experiences are enriching. This is possible, even for those living with a medical condition. The key lies in our life scripts and what we have decided to believe about ourselves.

Below are a few life scripts that many people have that do more harm than good. If you notice that you have created some of these scripts in your own life, don't fret. Remember that you can always rewrite your life story and your experience living with ADHD.

Script: I always put other people first.

This script may stem from one's upbringing or their expected social roles; whatever the root, it is a common script for those living with ADHD. By putting other people first, it almost takes the spotlight away from you and having to express who you are. You may be uncomfortable speaking about your condition with others or allowing others to see beneath your visage. This script is fueled by the assumption that if you please others, you will be accepted, liked, and treated "normal". The issue with this script is that it negates the fact that you also have needs which are valid, important, and that should be supported, too.

Investing in yourself isn't selfish, self-indulgent, or a display of arrogance. Similarly, telling others no isn't a form of rejection or disapproval of who they are nor is it diminishing their needs in any way. Sometimes, saying no is simply drawing the line between help that is empowering to both of you and help that only benefits the receiver while compromising your own well-being.

Script: Bad things always happen to me.

People who have this script usually possess an immense fear of failure. Moreover, they can be perfectionists at work or overly extend themselves in relationships, which places them in danger of being hurt or having their high expectations unmet.

The underlying belief of this script is that mistakes can lead to harmful consequences and, therefore, must be avoided at all costs. People who have this script find it difficult to relax their harsh self-imposed standards or let themselves off the hook. Usually, the internal backlash and self-criticism that they allow within themselves are far more severe than backlash received from others.

The danger of this script is seen in how it stifles creativity and makes people afraid of trying out new things that are outside of their comfort zones. Conversely, it tends to lead to a feeling of being under pressure constantly.

Script: I am never good enough.

People who feel like they are never good enough can display it publicly through suffering depression or anxiety. Alternatively, it can be disguised in phrases like, "I'm only as good as my last project/achievement." Initially, the disguise seems positive; I mean, who wouldn't want to strive to continually better themselves? Nonetheless, this constant seeking and striving hides an emptiness inside that can never truly be filled with any achievement.

The only way to really feel that you are enough is to accept yourself as you are and know that you are already a valuable and respectable individual.

Reader Task: The Acceptance Speech

Take a moment to reflect on something about yourself that makes you feel ashamed, guilty, insecure, or not good enough. Maybe it is something related to your personality, behavioral patterns, abilities/inabilities, relationships with others, or your medical condition. Once you have identified something (or a few things), write them down and describe how they make you feel using keywords. Does this thing make you feel sad? Embarrassed? Angry? Confused? Hopeless? Try to write as truthfully as you can, keeping in mind that no one else will see what you write.

The second part of this exercise is about writing a self-acceptance letter addressed to yourself. In the letter, you have an opportunity to express compassion, understanding, and acceptance toward yourself for the parts of yourself or your life that you dislike. As you write your self-acceptance letter, use the following list as a guideline:

1. Imagine a person who loves you unconditionally and accepts you for who you are (this person may be real or fictional). What would they have to say about the part of you that you dislike?

2. As you write, remind yourself that no one is perfect; everyone has flaws. Think about the millions of people in the world who are also dealing with the same situations as you.

3. Reflect on how your upbringing, family environment, or genes (external factors) may have, in some way, contributed to this negative quality about yourself.

4. In a very compassionate manner, ask yourself if there are things you can do or measures you can take to better cope with this negative quality. Remind yourself of how constructive and positive strategies can make you feel happier, healthier, and more fulfilled.

5. Once you have written the letter, put it down for a few hours or a couple of days. When you return to it, read it aloud to yourself, taking regular pauses to truly absorb what you have written. It may be useful to keep the letter in a place where you can easily reach it. You may want to refer back to it when you feel like you're under pressure, challenged by social stigmas, or feeling insecure again about the same things. This letter will serve as a perfect reminder to accept yourself for who you are and be kind to your journey.

Chapter 2:

It's Not You, It's Your

Treatment

Soon after being diagnosed with ADHD, patients are given a list of possible remedies to calm the symptoms. A doctor's favorite treatment will involve a cocktail of medicines that promise to give you a "normal" life. Many times—perhaps due to the initial shock or numbness after receiving a diagnosis—patients don't question whether drugs are the safest and healthiest intervention for regulating their symptoms. They mindlessly accept that for the rest of their lives they will live on drugs to feel normal.

For many years, medication has been seen as the answer to treating ADHD. Ask any doctor and they will tell you that it is the best option for regulating symptoms. The popularity of prescriptions like Ritalin and Adderall have also led to the misuse and abuse of ADHD medicine, similarly to how energy drinks have been incorrectly used to boost concentration or work longer hours. The abuse of ADHD medication has led to a public mockery of this serious medical condition and to questions regarding whether ADHD medicine truly works or if it is merely an excuse to self-medicate.

What many people don't realize about ADHD medicine is that it doesn't work for everyone. In other words, ADHD medication is not a miracle drug. Even when they do work for patients, they don't eliminate or permanently remove all symptoms. Some patients find that for the first few months or years their medication works well, but without any notice, it will suddenly stop working. Other patients find that ever since they started using ADHD medication, their symptoms have only gotten worse and more pronounced in their daily lives.

One study found that 30% of children who had ADHD didn't respond to stimulants or couldn't tolerate the devastating side-effects (Moleculera Labs, 2020). The same study found that 1 in every 3 adults diagnosed with ADHD did not improve their symptoms on standard ADHD medication (Moleculera Labs, 2020). While medication can improve one's attention and concentration, it generally doesn't help with other significant symptoms like disorganization, poor time management, procrastination, and forgetfulness—the bread and butter issues that cause a lot of challenges for adults with ADHD.

Another concern with standard ADHD medication is that it is a hit or miss. What I mean by this is that everybody responds differently to it. There are some who have experienced dramatic improvements while others have seen little to no improvements at all. The side-effects of the medications also differ for each individual. Some may never experience any side-effects while others notice a decline in health because of them.

Since everyone responds differently, it can be exhausting hopping from one drug to the next trying to find one appropriate for you. In this search for the perfect drug, it is rare for people to pause, take a second to breathe, and ask themselves, "Do I really need this?"

The Worst Drug Side-Effect: The Loss of Spontaneous Expression

Psychiatrist Peter Breggin studied the effects of stimulant drugs like Ritalin on the brain. The results were so disturbing that they led him to write an article protesting against the drugging of children and warning counselors and psychologists of the unspoken damages stimulant drugs can cause.

In his research, Breggin found that stimulant drugs suppress unwanted behaviors that are deemed inappropriate in a classroom, workplace, or controlled family environment. That wasn't all, though. He also found that stimulants lead to obsessive-compulsive behaviors that are desired in those same environments.

When stimulant drugs were tested on animals, a sudden shift in behavior was observed. The animals lost their natural spontaneity to move about, explore, exercise, socialize, innovate, and play. Suppressing their natural spontaneity with stimulant drugs turned these spirited animals into docile and manageable creatures.

Similar to children, animals aren't fans of routine, rigid tasks, or mundane activities. However, stimulant drugs enforced these controlled and rigid behaviors in them, producing what is known as *perseveration* in animal research. In human research, the same behavior is known as "obsessive-compulsive", or "over-focused", behavior.

For instance, when an animal was given stimulant drugs, they would sit quietly in their cage, preoccupied with behaviors like compulsive grooming, chewing on their paws, or staring into open space. In this state, the animals are more submissive or controllable and can be easily handled. Breggin found that the effects of stimulant drugs on children are identical to those found in animals. In other words, the biochemical or neurological effect was exactly the same. Many times, adverse drug reactions when taking stimulant medication can be mistaken as improving one's symptoms and behaviors when, in fact, it is doing the opposite.

For example, some may believe the adverse drug reaction of over-focusing is a positive behavior to display, especially for someone with ADHD who finds maintaining focus challenging. Over-focusing may be seen as a strength at work, helping you meet deadlines and participate more effectively in meetings and so on. However, too much focus can be harmful to your well-being. Over-focusing can drain your brain, turning you into an apathetic person and preventing you from seeing and experiencing everything around you. Abusing your brain's capacity to focus can lead to chronic fatigue which, over time, impacts your productivity and ability to perform at your peak.

Your brain only has so much energy, and when it is running on empty, it cannot stretch itself any further. It is important to have time off to allow your brain to unfocus for a while. This will ensure that when it is active, you are operating at your optimum capacity.

Besides suppressing spontaneous behaviors and causing more obsessive-compulsive or over-focused behaviors, stimulant drugs can also lead to emotional issues. When the dosage of ADHD medication is too high, for instance, it can cause both children and adults to appear "spacey" or "zombie-like". Sometimes, they can also display behaviors that are out of their character like being tearful or irritable.

Swanson and his co-scientists (1992) investigated the emotional turmoil that ADHD medication drug methylphenidate had on patients. They found that beyond the drug-induced compliant behavior, patients became isolated, withdrawn, and somber. They noticed that this somberness eventually led to social isolation, with patients preferring to spend time alone as opposed to interacting with others.

Many researchers have mentioned that this zombie-like effect brought upon by stimulant drugs causes patients to lose touch with what is happening in the present. This drugged state is not therapeutic, as some would suggest. Rather, it is an act of theft, stealing the possibility of its users experiencing and living life completely in the moment.

The Link Between ADHD Medication and Anxiety

ADHD medication can sometimes make matters worse rather than better. Some of the common side-effects of ADHD drugs that many people deal with include insomnia, a loss of appetite, and having tics. However, even more common is the side-effect that most of us dread: anxiety. These are not issues that anyone should tolerate, especially as a result of medicine that is supposed to enhance the quality of one's life.

It's not uncommon for those living with ADHD to also suffer from anxiety, whether it is part of the symptoms from the medication or due to a full-blown anxiety disorder. In fact, a study found that 30 to 40% of people living with ADHD have an anxiety disorder which may or may not include obsessive-compulsive disorder, phobias, social anxiety, and panic disorder. In some cases, the symptoms that come with ADHD can cause anxiety. For instance, you might miss an important deadline at work, forget to respond to an email, or act impulsively and put yourself in a dangerous situation. Even the constant fear that you might forget something is enough to cause an anxious behavioral response.

Naturally, people with ADHD (both those receiving treatment and otherwise) tend to be more emotionally sensitive, which can lead to them feeling things more deeply and being more impacted by shifting environmental factors around them. Many times, stimulant medication can exacerbate the anxiety that already exists within patients. For instance, stimulant drugs can produce a physical sensation of heart palpitations, dry mouth, shortness of breath, and they can activate the fight-or-flight response. The presence of anxiety can even compromise treatment because of how paralyzing it can be to feel threatened by your environment.

Usually, patients with anxiety tend to get stuck in their old ways and are less likely to try new things like alternative treatments for fear that these alternative treatments won't work out for them. Adults who have ADHD along with an anxiety disorder may find it challenging to fully function in their everyday lives. This is because anxiety usually takes a person out of the present moment by causing them to think back on past memories or forward to future events.

The inability to be present in the moment causes a lack of environmental awareness—a lack of being aware of the responsibilities and choices that are presented to you here and now, which could benefit you and promote good health.

The combination of ADHD symptoms and an anxiety disorder may lead to one feeling a constant threat in their lives. This can make it difficult for them to organize information in a rational and productive way and see the bigger picture of their lives and their current situation. For example, you may be feeling a continuous threat that your ADHD symptoms will cause you humiliation in public, and this threat may increase your levels of anxiety in public spaces or when you are interacting with others. The longer it continues to exist, the more debilitating your anxiety will be. At times, it may cause you to withdraw socially and prefer being alone or with people you are accustomed to.

You don't have to settle for a life where you are constantly anxious. A life of neverending worry and fear of everyday situations does not have to be your normal. I guarantee that it's possible to treat anxiety in a way that doesn't involve forcing more drugs down your throat.

However, before I present you with natural treatments for ADHD, it is important for you to understand the type of anxiety that you have so that you know what to focus on during treatment and to effectively reduce any ADHD symptoms that are associated with that type of anxiety. Take a look at the description for each type of anxiety below, and try to think of your own anxiety woes.

1.   Generalized Anxiety Disorder (GAD)

Generalized anxiety disorder is typically characterized by ongoing worry and a fear of everyday situations. It interferes with your daily routines, hindering the way you work, study, or engage in relationships with others. People with GAD will expect the worst possible outcome, even when there isn't a reasonable cause for concern.

2. Social Anxiety

Social anxiety refers to the extreme fear of being criticized, judged, or humiliated by others in a social setting or performance-related situation. Even though the sufferer may recognize that their fear is exaggerated or irrational, they are still extremely afraid of embarrassment or social rejection.

3. Post-Traumatic Stress Disorder (PTSD)

Post-traumatic stress disorder is a condition that happens in people who have experienced a natural disaster, violence, a serious accident, the death of a loved one, prolonged sickness, or any other life-threatening situation in their lives.

4. Obsessive-Compulsive Disorder (OCD)

Obsessive-compulsive disorder compels sufferers to experience intrusive or worrisome thoughts that replay in their minds obsessively. These thoughts often cause them to perform behaviors and routines repetitively or ritualistically in an attempt to ease their anxiety.

5. Phobias

Phobias are irrational fears that cause sufferers to make a conscious effort to avoid certain places, situations, or things. Some examples of phobias include animals, heights, germs, public transportation, thunder, and medical procedures.

It is always recommended to treat ADHD and anxiety simultaneously. Generally, when ADHD symptoms are handled in a healthy way, anxiety tends to be reduced. Conversely, as the levels of anxiety are decreased, ADHD symptoms lessen gradually as well. Since stimulant drugs may aggravate one's anxiety and cause other harmful side-effects, it is ideal for those with ADHD to look for healthier treatment options that will reduce the symptoms of ADHD without bringing upon more psychological issues.

While medication offers immediate relief from some of these symptoms, it also creates dependency, and this means that you will never truly get to live a life free from drugs. This dependency also causes you to settle for whatever side-effects may come along with them, hopelessly consenting to the health risks associated with stimulant medication. Alternative treatments are available, and it is my hope to share some of these with you throughout this book.

Outside the Pill Bottle: CBT for Adult ADHD

Even though medications are perceived as the frontline treatment for adults with ADHD, there has been plenty of research to suggest that medication alone cannot sufficiently treat many of the symptoms that develop as a result of this medical condition. For instance, drugs cannot effectively treat the psychological effects experienced as a result of living with ADHD. This should be alarming, seeing that most people who are diagnosed with the condition are presented with at least one other psychiatric diagnosis, the most common of these being anxiety, depression, and substance addiction.

While medication can improve one's concentration, it does very little to enhance daily functioning or one's development and life experiences. Where the effectiveness of medication ends, the promise and benefits of psychotherapy begin. One of the other available treatments for ADHD is psychosocial treatment. It is available in various models that are adapted to meet the needs of adults with ADHD.

You may be wondering what psychosocial treatments offer that medical treatments don't. The main difference between the two is that medical treatments target specific ADHD-related symptoms whereas psychosocial treatments target functional impairments, helping patients discover, develop, and implement healthy coping strategies in their daily lives. The most studied psychosocial treatment is a model of psychotherapy known as cognitive-behavioral therapy (CBT).

What differentiates CBT from other forms of psychotherapy is the emphasis it places on the role of cognitions—images, automatic thoughts, and belief systems—and behaviors. CBT addresses emotions by targeting problematic thinking and behavioral patterns which are the root cause for why many seek treatment. Originally, CBT was a treatment used to treat depression, mood swings, and anxiety, but within the past decade, many clinical studies have been conducted that are working on ways to modify CBT to cope with symptoms associated with adult ADHD.

CBT has been found time and again to be a great ADHD treatment when used in combination with other treatments. It helps individuals with ADHD address the impairments and difficulties associated with the diagnosis. This is done by offering coping strategies to adjust negative thoughts and behavioral patterns. Facing these thoughts and behaviors may help to effectively eliminate pessimism, self-criticism, anxiety, and feelings of frustration and replace them with strategies for managing time, planning tasks, and working through negative emotions.

A common example of how CBT works can be seen in a case study of a patient who arrives late to their first CBT session, mentioning that "poor time management" is one of their goals for CBT. The therapist would use this real-life scenario to expose components of the problem in order to help the patient understand how ADHD (and other related factors) may be contributing to the development and maintenance of some of their problems—in this case, poor time management. Having gained an understanding of what, how, and why these problems continue to manifest, the patient would then be given suggestions, ideas, and strategies for coping and improving the severity of the problem.

Another great benefit of CBT is that treatment is personalized for each individual, because every patient suffers from different mental and emotional issues at varying degrees. Since treatment is personalized to each individual's circumstance, it improves the success rate of each intervention and ensures that the coping strategies and skills are relevant and useful.

To continue with the same case study mentioned above, a CBT therapist may find that the patient's poor time management is caused by a few or all of the factors listed below:

- Not being good at keeping a daily schedule or planner (hence forgetting the time of the appointment)
- Being disorganized (the patient may have misplaced the piece of paper with the address details of the therapy session)

- Poor problem-solving abilities (the patient may not have known how to think on the spot about ways to find the contact details of the therapist online or reschedule the appointment)
- Not being good at planning (the patient may not have had a realistic timeframe for leaving their house, getting on public transportation, and reaching the appointment room)
- Becoming overly focused on other distractions (the patient may have watched TV or been on the computer for longer than they should have, thus running late for the appointment)

Each of these possible causes of poor time management offers the patient an opportunity for change. As every difficulty associated with ADHD is discussed and analyzed in context to the patient's daily life, recurring themes will emerge and a number of coping skills will be shared. These coping skills can be learned and applied to various areas of the patient's daily routine to improve their overall daily functioning.

CBT does a thorough job of reaching the root of the problem and coming up with personalized solutions to improve cognitive abilities and behaviors. However, it would be erroneous of us to assume that CBT is an easy or quick fix. The skills that are discussed must be implemented by the patient if they desire to experience any change. Otherwise, the therapy session becomes like any other general therapy which won't necessarily target symptoms related to ADHD.

Cognitive-Behavioral Therapy in Action

One of the most common issues experienced by adults with ADHD is procrastination. While most patients suffer from this problem, cognitive-behavioral therapy would address it differently with each patient. This is because every individual's struggle with procrastination is unique. Once a patient identifies procrastination as their goal for CBT treatment, they are encouraged by the therapist to share recent examples of this procrastination in their daily routine.

For example, the patient may have recently procrastinated filling out important administration forms. The therapist would then assess the patient's relationship with the task. He or she would break the task down into components in order to organize it into actionable steps (also known as chunking). After presenting the task in steps, both the patient and therapist would identify any potential barriers or deterrents that could influence the patient's ability to follow through with each step.

Another important part of this discovery process is explicitly looking at the patient's cognitive and emotional reactions when they speak about the task or the prospect of engaging with the task again. Some of the common questions that therapists will ask patients at this juncture include:

- "What are the thoughts going through your mind about performing this task?"
- "What emotions rise up within you when you think about performing this task?"

- "What does your body experience when you are faced with this task?"

The purpose of asking these questions is to assess the significance of negative thoughts and emotions that may also be contributing to the issue of procrastination. These questions will reveal the patient's fight or flight behaviors and rationalizations, an example of which being telling oneself they will first eat and check their mail before sitting down to fill out administration forms.

You will find that CBT interventions work similarly to the way executive functions are designed to operate. Executive functions are those cognitive skills that are indispensable for self-control and regulating behaviors. They help people plan, organize, and manage their time and energy to fulfill tasks that may not necessarily offer an immediate reward but tend to offer long-term benefits.

Various CBT Intervention Approaches

There are numerous CBT intervention approaches that promote cognitive and emotional improvements for adults with ADHD. For instance, one approach that can be useful for patients is the use of sessions as a form of prolongation. Prolongation is simply an in-depth and extended reflection on an experience that allows individuals to analyze all sides of a situation and find meaning. In CBT sessions, prolongation allows patients to assess the situation, consider available options, plan a course of action, and implement the plan effectively. This provides the necessary support for adults with ADHD, who tend to delay an action or plan that is not imminent, minimize its significance or make a quick decision about a course of action without carefully considering the options available.

Another CBT intervention approach is problem management. While it is natural for all human beings to face difficult problems in their lives, adults with ADHD may find problem-solving daunting. During CBT sessions, therapists will address individual problems and coping topics and strategies to go through each step of problem management and plan for possible barriers to a smooth follow-through.

Interventions can also focus on providing psychoeducation as part of building a patient's mental framework. In fact, sometimes the first step in any cognitive intervention is to gain an accurate assessment of the patient's ADHD, as the diagnosis offers possible reasons as to why a patient feels, thinks, or acts in the ways that they do. Many times, if this step is missed, cognitive and behavioral symptoms that are ADHD-related may be passed off as being a character flaw or an ingrained self-defeating behavior.

Psychoeducation is also vital because it offers patients an in-depth understanding and recognition of the impact of ADHD on their lives. For instance, adults with ADHD have a difficult time creating systems and routines in their lives. However, this isn't because they don't know what needs to be done, but rather it is due to difficulty implementing the change. Interventions that follow tend to be more effective because they build upon the mental framework that has already been established in the minds of patients.

A crucial component of psychoeducation is discussing issues related to environmental engineering. Environmental engineering is the process of setting up one's environment (living, working, and studying settings) to make them more ADHD-friendly. By this, I mean creating systems in one's environment that help to bypass the effects of executive dysfunction. Some examples of proactive systems include the following: reducing any possible distractions in work or study settings, organizing automatic payment plans, using a daily planner, and so on.

While many of the coping strategies and environmental engineering suggestions won't be new to patients, the purpose of introducing them again is to ensure that they are implemented in the most efficient and manageable way possible (planning for possible obstacles that may interfere with follow-through).

The focus on implementation is quite different from a goal-oriented approach. Goal-oriented approaches assume that a person can hold in their minds the desired goal that will drive specific behaviors necessary to achieve the outcome. Of course, this is challenging for a person living with ADHD, who finds it difficult to follow through on such goals. The implementation focus, on the other hand, identifies and isolates important decision-making milestones in targeted behaviors, such as getting started on a project or gathering information for a report. Prolongation is then used to explain the significance of the situation, construct a meaningful plan of action, and review the patient's motivation to follow through with the prospective plan.

Chapter 3:

The Cure Lies in the Body

The body knows how to heal itself. More and more, many people are coming to the realization that healing is a holistic process. You are happiest, healthiest, and the most filled with vitality when your physical body, mind, and emotions are in perfect alignment. The true definition of healing is to make something whole. This means that true healing cannot only happen at one level, but must occur on all three levels—the physical, mental, and emotional levels.

When a patient seeks to heal a mental condition such as ADHD, they can trust that their body knows how to heal itself. All they are required to do is get out of the way, listen to the information being given by their body, and allow it to heal. The ADHD symptoms that you would usually associate with pain and suffering are simply your body's way of showing you that there is an imbalance that needs to be corrected. If everyone saw the symptoms as being this straightforward, there wouldn't be a need for heavy doses of medicine to try to get to the root of the issue.

Medication is not skin deep. It can only address what a patient experiences on one level. Sometimes, physical symptoms can be addressed through medication, exercise, or surgery, but the issue will not have been addressed in its entirety; the mental and emotional consequences of the issue must also receive attention in order for holistic healing to take place.

The more society has progressed, the less people have held onto the practice of listening to their bodies and their intuitive minds. If only we could take a few moments to sit down, turn off the TV, and rest when we feel tired or express our anger, sadness, or confusion naturally instead of suppressing what needs to be released. But the message we receive from the media, our communities, and corporate institutions is to stay composed at all times. In other words, we are told it is shameful to cry, show frustration, or admit that we are stressed and under extreme pressure. All of the unnatural cures or remedies that patients with ADHD are given are engineered to instill a composed, "everything is fine with me" image while deep inside, things are not fine.

Healing that occurs on one level and neglects the others causes an individual to feel disconnected and fragmented. In one part of their lives, they are free and healthy, but in another, they feel out of control and emotionally bankrupt. You might have a healthy habit of drinking green juices and exercising daily, but as soon as you neglect your mental and emotional health, you are less likely to feel fulfilled and whole. Since the cure lies in the body, the solution to all of your physical, mental, and emotional issues must lie in the body, too. This means that everywhere you walk, you are carrying answers within you to effectively solve some of the mysterious symptoms you have dealt with all of your life. To find these solutions, it only takes one simple action: listen.

When you listen to what you are sensing intuitively within you and how you are feeling in various circumstances, you come closer and closer to realizing the root of the issue and subsequently have a clear idea of how to resolve it.

Recovery Is Possible

You can recover from mental illness. If you find it difficult to take my word for it, perhaps a research study undertaken by the National Empowerment Center will be more convincing. The study conducted in-depth interviews with people battling schizophrenia and found that it was possible for these individuals to regain prominent roles in society and independently run their own lives. This group was able to heal from their mental illness, and they continued to heal emotionally, as well. They gradually got off medication and instead opted for holistic health and peer support as ways of continuing to take positive steps toward healing.

This study was consistent with the one undertaken in this country by Dr. Courtenay Harding and colleagues, and in Europe by Dr. Manfred Bleuler and Dr. Luc Ciompi. These two additional studies showed that within a 20- to 30-year period, it was possible for a majority of people to completely recover from even the most critical of mental illnesses.

In spite of this evidence, there are many individuals, doctors, and therapists who believe that once someone is diagnosed with a mental disorder, they can never fully recover. Even most rehabilitation professionals will argue that mental illness is a permanent life sentence. I believe without a shadow of a doubt that fear is a significant factor in perpetuating this myth of no recovery. Those people who are labeled as "normal" fear entering the realms of "madness", and those who have been labeled "mad" fear being overcome by what many believe has no cure. This fear also creates separateness or an "other".

People who are labeled as normal are comfortable thinking those who have been diagnosed with a mental or emotional disorder have a genetically-based brain malfunction that they don't have. If more professionals and individuals spoke about the possibility of recovery from mental illness, the "other" would disappear and there would be no need for prolonged use of medication. In fact, if more people realized that recovery was possible, they would see that anyone can be labeled as mentally ill and fully heal from it, too.

Dissolving the Pain-Body

You may not know it, but you have old unresolved emotions within you. Everyone does. These emotions are an accumulation of painful life experiences that were never addressed or accepted in the moments they arose. This left behind an energy form of emotional pain that lingers in your body. This energy is combined with others of emotional pain collected through various life experiences.

The end result is a "pain-body", an entity of energy within you that carries a record of emotional pain. You may not notice the presence of this pain-body on a normal day or during your daily routines—it rarely interrupts routines or programmed ways of thinking. Nevertheless, it will arise (or become triggered) when a situation, person, or task sets off a strong emotion. At this point, the pain-body will take over your mind and attempt to make sense of an experience which is presented as a threat to it. Your internal dialogue, which can be negative at times, becomes the voice of this pain-body talking to you internally.

You will know when the pain-body is speaking because it can only bring up old painful emotions or old dysfunctional behaviors. Every belief, opinion, judgment, or interpretation that it has about you, your situation, or other people will be grossly distorted by old emotional pain.

It is so easy for people to identify with the pain-body and believe its justifications when they are unaware of what it is or that it has taken over their mind. They end up embracing negative thoughts as their own and settling for the disempowering suggestions or ideas made by this pain-body. Once the pain-body is active, it grows in energy and thrives on self-defeating actions, words, and thoughts. After it has grown considerably in energy, people find that they cannot seem to stop thinking anxious or discouraging thoughts throughout the day and night. Soon, physical effects such as exhaustion, overthinking, worry, or insomnia start showing up as an indication of a much deeper and more serious problem.

If you think your pain-body is only after you, think again. Remember that at its purest form it is energy and, therefore, it can be transferred between people. There are times when your pain-body will desire to feed on somebody else's reaction to trigger them into activating their own pain-body and start a larger chain reaction. If you live with your romantic partner or family, your pain-body will seek to provoke them enough to trigger a negative response. If your partner or family members are not aware of this game of great deception, they will react, and the chain reaction officially begins.

Both your and your partner's pain-bodies are now fully active and feeding on each other in order to survive. After a few days of feeding (drama, arguments, tension, etc.), both pain-bodies will be satisfied and go back into a dormant state. This is typically when you look at your partner and ask them, "What was all of that fighting about?" On some occasions, you may not even remember what incited the conflict or why it turned ugly so quickly. However, what you don't yet realize is that this pain-body will revisit or become active again when it is triggered—and the horror of past emotional pain will haunt you or your family once more.

How to Heal the Pain-Body

One of my favorite quotes by Eckhart Tolle is this: "Rather than being your thoughts and emotions, be the awareness behind them." Your feelings and how you think create a narrative that you end up living in. When this narrative is dark, hopeless, and full of trouble, you can expect to live under a constant dark cloud. There are some who will ignorantly believe that this cloud must be the grim reality of living with a medical condition, but it is not. Remember that at the end of the day, ADHD is only a diagnosis. How this diagnosis affects you or changes your life has a lot to do with the lens through which you perceive it.

There are some people living with ADHD who feel completely debilitated by their diagnosis, and there are others who are flourishing in their professional and private lives. Is this because the severity of ADHD is different for these individuals? No. They live completely different lives because of what they choose to see, believe, think, and feel about themselves, their lives, and the world around them.

Healing the pain-body doesn't require any external intervention. For the first time, you will learn how healing resonates from within. It makes sense why healing of any kind would resonate from inside yourself. Take a moment, and assess how pain (whether physical, mental, or emotional) develops. Does it come as a result of an external or internal reaction? Do you become hurt because of what is done to you or because of how you feel about what is done to you?

Perhaps we can take a quick look at the science of pain to point us toward a formidable conclusion. What we know as pain starts at the source of the injury, whether it is physical, emotional, or mental. The physical message from the injury passes from where the hurt took place and travels directly to the brain. It is only when the message reaches the brain that it is registered as the sensation of pain. The brain then takes it upon itself to create a memory of this sensation, store it for safekeeping (in case the injury occurs again), and send the message back to the area of injury. This detailed process happens within seconds but has lasting consequences, such as the development of a pain-body.

Instead of identifying with your injury or pain-body, you can become the awareness behind it. Pain doesn't have to be a threat once it is recognized and effectively dealt with. In fact, many times, when our bodies signal that we are in pain, all the pain is looking for is some recognition, and it will gently fade away. You can compassionately witness emotional energy from the past that is trying to get your attention so that it can come to full completion and be released. You can heal your pain-body by following the steps listed below:

1. **Catch the pain-body as it arises and is still in its inception.**

The pain-body will always arise as a negative, self-defeating, or worrisome thought or feeling that originates from your past. Catching the pain-body as it activates within you will ensure that you stop it in its tracks before further injury is caused. For instance, you can catch feelings of unhappiness, insecurity, worthlessness, anger, or any other similar thought before it fully forms. This could mean starting to listen attentively to the internal dialogue taking place in your mind throughout the day. Notice the times of the day or which tasks trigger your pain-body and activate these negative thoughts and feelings.

Anger, for example, may start as irritation that progressively becomes deeper the more the pain-body grows within you. Negative thoughts about being worthless may begin as a feeling of loneliness that progressively becomes more negative. Other times, the pain-body can be activated by dark desires that come into your mind to either hurt yourself, hurt others, or create unnecessary drama in your environment.

2. Observe your pain-body without thinking.

Step two may sound strange. I mean, how can you focus on anything without thinking about it? Observing here means becoming more alert about the sensations, thoughts, and feelings flowing through your body as the pain-body develops. In other words, it requires you to sit with the uncomfortable feeling and watch it as it tries to control your mind, body, and emotions. Observe where the pain-body travels; is it to your head or heart? Observe how it changes your body language; do you become more rigid and withdrawn from others? Observe how it changes the quality of your thoughts and your overall mood.

It is also important to observe your resistance to feeling your emotional pain. Observe how you try to suppress it with another thought or feeling or how you pretend like it doesn't exist. Lastly, observe how easy it is to identify with this pain and to embrace it as being true for you in this moment. Pay attention to how comfortable this pain is to come into your body and make itself at home. Observe your natural tendency to make other people or other circumstances responsible for this emotional pain by assuming the role of victim, passing blame onto others, and making excuses.

3. **Cultivate and direct unconditional love and attention to your pain-body.**

After identifying and observing your pain-body, you are now in a position to cultivate and direct unconditional love and attention to it. I'm sure you have heard people speaking about accepting your flaws and how this is supposed to be a pathway to peace, love, and freedom.

While I agree with this suggestion, I find that many times, we are not told how to locate these flaws within us and how to transfer acceptance. The hard part is finding the pain-body and knowing what it is, where it comes from, and what its intentions are in your body. Cultivating and directing love and attention are easier because these actions come so naturally to you. The love and attention you will focus on your pain-body can be found overflowing within you.

If you are not used to directing love and attention toward yourself, you will find this step awkward, to say the least. However, it is still natural. Focus loving attention on your negative emotional pain. It may help to smile as you think about your pain-body or gently repeat compassionate words like "hope", "kindness", "love", or "peace".

4. Express your emotional pain in a meaningful way.

We know that hiding emotional pain only fuels the hurt and causes it to seek our attention even more. When loving attention is focused on the pain, we are forced to validate its presence, and it gradually subsides. Nevertheless, there is more that you and I can do to make sure that we learn from our uninvited guest and grow in the understanding of ourselves and how deeply we feel. We can express our experience with the pain-body through various creative and meaningful avenues.

For instance, those who like to draw or paint can illustrate the experience of feeling the pain-body activate, how it became a strong negative emotion, and the transformation that took place when love and attention were given to it. Other ways of expressing the experience with your pain-body are through journaling, recording yourself detailing the experience, dancing, playing music, or exercising.

Reducing Anxiety Through Self-Awareness

Being a person who feels every emotion so intensely is not easy. While your intelligent nervous system allows you to feel a range of pleasurable sensations and feelings, it is also programmed to sense possible threats in your environment and sound the alarm when you are in perceived danger. But what happens when your nervous system perceives even the most natural or circumstantial situation as a threat? The short answer is you become anxious, even when the situation isn't life-threatening.

I have heard many people with anxiety express their desire to "get rid of anxiety" because it is ruining their lives. I am hesitant to agree with them on this sentiment because I believe that it is normal and healthy to feel anxious to some degree at certain times. For example, if you are about to take a test, go to a job interview, go on a date, or perform in front of an audience, having anxiety is normal and part of the experience. This kind of positive anxiety reminds you that you are stepping out of your comfort zone, doing something brave, and creating new experiences. In other words, it is confirmation that you are alive!

Nevertheless, the negative form of anxiety is that which sounds fake warning signals to the brain when in reality, there is no threat in sight. Imagine how it feels when someone plays a prank on you but uses a serious crisis to make the joke more believable. Your mind immediately believes it to be true and your body starts preparing its survival instinct to attack, defend, act, or withdraw yourself from the crisis. Now, let's say after a few minutes of this running joke, the individual says "I'm only joking!" You might give a great sigh of relief, but your body is still in survival mode and will be for the next few hours.

Negative anxiety has the same effect on those who are triggered by situations, tasks, or events that are not actually threatening. Several alarms are sounded every day, signaling danger in everyday routines and functions. When the nervous system is constantly engaged and activated by fake warning signs, it may lead those affected to have enraged outbursts, have the desire to avoid social situations, and become immobile or apathetic. This results in a disconnection with the world around them, social awkwardness, and a deep feeling of isolation or loneliness which can cause further emotional and mental pain.

Self-Awareness: The Path to Mental Well-Being

Self-awareness is one of those psychological terms that has been thrown around in every conversation and, at times, has been misused. At its core, self-awareness is a powerful skill that can potentially transform how you see and feel about yourself within the context of the environment around you. One way of defining self-awareness is to say that it is the practice of taking a step back and observing your thoughts and feelings as they take place in a non-judgmental and non-interfering way. It includes something as simple as paying attention to how you feel when you are preparing to go to work, when you encounter certain people, or when you are faced with certain challenges.

Those with high levels of self-awareness can take it a step further and observe how their changing thoughts throughout the day impact their emotional state, motivation, and behaviors. For example, it could be a Monday and the thought of going to work may cause the person to feel discouraged, leading to a delay or procrastination of tasks such as getting ready and leaving the house in time.

Another way of looking at self-awareness is to see it as a way of shining a light on the parts of your internal world that may otherwise be hidden or go unnoticed. The awareness of these "less glamorous" parts of yourself is the first step to healing and growth. After all, it is impossible to change something that you are unaware of.

Growth comes as a result of your understanding that you are not the voice of your mind, but instead, you are the one who observes the shenanigans that your mind is up to. It takes courage to come to this point, because the act of standing "outside" of your own mind may feel uncomfortable or, in extreme cases, confrontational. It's like watching a recording of yourself during your most embarrassing or cringe-worthy moments, something that nobody willingly signs up for. Nevertheless, this self-awareness is necessary because it will gradually shift your focus away from what's happening in your environment, the crises at work, or the daily struggles of living with ADHD, and place the focus on yourself.

The whole point of self-awareness is not necessarily to love what you see (it is not a form of self-love). It is important that you realize this from the onset so that you are not disappointed when you see an ugly habit or behavior continually being repeated in your life. True self-awareness involves a level of detachment from your own mind and emotions so that you can clearly see what is happening without any biases, defensive behavior, or subjectivity.

Therefore, you must accept that there will be thoughts and feelings within you that you will not like at all. The positive side to all of this observation is that you will discover other parts of yourself that you haven't witnessed before. This is because alongside your fears, anxieties, and self-defeating behaviors there are just as many (if not more) of your natural strengths, talents, and skills that should also be noticed and given much-needed attention. This means that you will see confusing and dark parts of yourself while simultaneously celebrating your natural creativity and hidden talents. If you haven't figured it out by now, human beings are naturally this complicated.

As you become more acquainted with these dark parts of yourself, the voice of your inner critic may arise and cause you to feel shameful or guilty about some of the thoughts, emotions, or behaviors you exhibit. For instance, you may find yourself saying "I wish I didn't blow up like that", or "I don't like that I spoke in that manner." The inner critic feeds off of shame, regret, and guilt. At best, these strong emotions could awaken your pain-body.

The most effective way to address the voice of the inner critic is to simply observe it without identifying with its words, attitude, and beliefs. Similarly to how you observe your pain-body as it tries to expand within you, observe these critical thinking patterns and notice the agenda behind them. For instance, ask yourself if these thoughts are trying to discourage you from taking positive action, becoming more social, or stepping out of your comfort zone. Remember to remain non-judgmental and detached from these thoughts, and focus love and attention on them until they dissipate.

Self-Awareness and Self-Compassion

Another way to counter the onslaught of the inner critic is to practice self-care and self-compassion as you observe your inner world. Practicing self-awareness without showing yourself compassion is a recipe for disaster and the quickest way to feel discouraged about what you see and feel. Taking an honest look at your life and how you think and feel requires you to accept that the negative thoughts and emotions that could arise are simply calling for love and attention. You will also need self-compassion to confront some of the contradictions existing within you.

The truth is that every one of us is a walking contradiction and can experience conflicting thoughts and emotions about any given situation or task. This is not hypocritical or a sign of being confused. Your perspective on the world isn't black or white (and I doubt any human experience can be this way). Instead, you and I perceive our environment in shades of grey.

For instance, you may be excited about the prospect of going to a music festival and watching your favorite band play, but at the same time unsettled by the thought that you will have to be amongst a crowd of people or fearful of the logistics of leaving your house, finding parking, walking to the arena, and making your way back home. Another example is when you find yourself feeling determined about an upcoming presentation at work while simultaneously feeling underqualified or less refined at presenting in front of your colleagues.

The more you observe these contradictions, the less of a stumbling block they will be to you proceeding with your desired action anyway. You may feel anxious about going to a music festival, but because you know this is a once in a lifetime opportunity, you will choose to be encompassed by the excitement of going instead of the present fears. Recognizing both emotions and thoughts will seem very liberating because you are not tied to any one of them, thus giving you the power to shape your experience and make decisions in spite of warning signals going off in your mind.

Another form of showing yourself compassion is being aware of the parts of yourself that are resistant to becoming self-aware. If you honestly believe that you can heal or experience positive change without any internal resistance, you can think again. It's the same as a dieter who is determined to lose weight on a new eating plan, and after a week finds it difficult to stay disciplined with their new lifestyle. Is it because they suddenly had a change of heart and don't desire to lose weight anymore? Absolutely not. They may still be determined to lose weight; however, they are facing internal resistance (in the form of triggering thoughts and emotions) which inhibit them from continuing to make positive progress.

You will face similar internal resistance. There will be a part of you that resists being more open and honest with yourself about how you think and feel. Your mind will try to protect you from opening a can of worms that it has spent years trying to conceal. You will feel overwhelmed or fearful of going deeper within yourself, and this is normal. When you feel an inner resistance or defensive behavior surfacing, simply observe the thoughts or sensations flowing through your body without getting involved. The more you sit with these anxious thoughts or feelings, the less of a hurdle or barrier they will become. It will also remind you that self-awareness is a journey and not a destination.

Reader Task: Re-Discovering Me

True self-awareness cannot be learned by reading a book. Rather, it is developed through regular self-reflection and using what you have learned about yourself to inform your decisions, behaviors, and interactions with others. Being aware of who you are can also help you identify your minor and major stressors at work, socially, and within intimate relationships. This information can be useful in building effective coping mechanisms that will help you manage stress in a more empowering way. Put simply, the more information you know about yourself, the better equipped you will be in adapting to various life changes.

Think about describing who you are to another person without mentioning any external factors such as your work, family, or friends. Focus specifically on yourself and share with this invisible person who you are and what you see, think, and feel about yourself. Tell them about your strengths, weaknesses, habits, and the things that make you the angriest and what makes you the happiest. You can write down your observations, record yourself speaking aloud, or use another creative medium to express (and keep a record) of what you share.

Below are a few questions that you can answer. They can help you get started on the task:

- What are your strengths and weaknesses? Think of three for each.
- What do you value the most?
- Differentiate between the things you can and cannot do by yourself.

- What feelings are you more aware of feeling strongly compared to other people?
- What are your triggers? This could be people and situations that provoke a negative emotional response or awaken your pain-body.
- How do you respond under stress? If you have a process for responding to stress, please explain it.
- How do the various roles you play in your life make you feel? This could be your role as a mother/father, sister/brother, wife/husband, friend, employee, etc.

Chapter 4:

The Mind-Body

Connection Explained

Julie is a well-educated, athletic, and social woman who may seem to many to have it all. She has a Ph.D., recently got engaged, and has a tight-knit circle of friends. Who wouldn't be envious of Julie, right?

Well, upon closer inspection of her life, Julie experiences challenges just like the rest of us. She has been diagnosed with type 2 diabetes, and the diagnosis hasn't brought much peace into her life. Even though Julie has the skills and talent to start her own business, she's anxious about how her medical condition may affect her entrepreneurial pursuits. The weight of pressure on her shoulders causes her to have emotional outbursts at work, snapping at her coworkers and feeling ashamed afterward. What's even more terrifying is that despite carefully monitoring her blood sugar, Julie finds herself in a coma once or twice a month.

Assessing Julie's experience, it is easy to see that she suffers from more than just diabetes. Despite her prosperous and healthy lifestyle, Julie's anxiety prevents her from paying attention to the signals that her body sends when her blood sugar is too low. This means that her diagnosis is not what's causing all of this pain, but rather her own behaviors of neglecting to listen to her body. If Julie were to pay attention to her body more, she would notice physical changes when her blood sugar starts dropping or when starting to feel anxious, stressed, and overwhelmed. This would prevent her from going into a diabetic coma, having emotional outbursts, and being fearful of using her education to progress in entrepreneurship.

Julie's story is a great example of the mind-body connection in action. The mind-body connection simply refers to the fact that your thoughts, emotions, behaviors, and beliefs can positively or negatively affect your biological functioning. In other words, the health of your body affects the health of your mind and vice versa. Your mind and body are constantly communicating with each other, creating a complex relationship between the two.

It is important not to confuse the word "mind" in mind-body connection with the brain. The mind refers to mental states, such as your thoughts, emotions, attitudes, beliefs, and images. The brain, on the other hand, is responsible for the intelligence that allows you to experience these mental states. Mental states can be completely conscious or subconscious, meaning that you may be aware of some of your thoughts and emotions, but not all of them. It also means that it is possible to have an emotional reaction to something and not understand why you decided to react in that particular way.

However, here's where mental states get interesting: every state that you experience (consciously or subconsciously) has physiology associated with it. This physiological reaction can be a positive or negative effect that is felt in the physical body. For example, the mental state of anxiety causes the body to release stress hormones. It is for this reason that many mind-body therapies emphasize raising clients' awareness to guide their mental states in a more empowering and less destructive direction.

The discovery of the mind-body connection is in no way new. Until 300 years ago, every system of medicine throughout various cultures and religions treated the mind and body as a whole. It was only during the 17th century that Western civilization began to view the mind and body as two separate entities. Doctors started to look at the body like a machine consisting of independent and replaceable parts without any connection whatsoever to the mind.

This Western view on the body had its fair share of benefits, helping to produce breakthroughs in surgeries, trauma care, and pharmaceuticals, but it also meant that there was less scientific inquiry into a human being's emotional and spiritual life and the innate ability for the body to heal itself.

By the 20th century, the Western viewpoint on healing started to change. This transformation was brought on by research studies looking at the mind-body connection and scientifically showing evidence of the complex links between the mind and the body.

ADHD and Sensory Processing Disorder

If you are living with ADHD, it is normal for you to also experience strong emotional reactions to things that others wouldn't find as upsetting or bothersome. It is natural for you to have a heightened and often exaggerated response to both positive and negative situations. You may also feel physical hypersensitivity to things like touch, sound, light, and even textures. For example, subtle sounds like the humming from an air conditioner or feeling the scratching from a tag on a shirt can become significant distractions for you. Instead of citing problems with inattention, you may suffer from over-focusing on smaller details, irritations, and sensations.

A person with ADHD hypersensitivity may also be called a highly sensitive person (HSP) who processes certain emotions and physical stimuli more intensely or attentively than others. They also tend to notice things within their surroundings in more detail, eventually leading to overstimulation and other ADHD-related symptoms. These symptoms may include extreme sensitivity to emotional or physical stimuli, an increased likelihood of asthma, allergies, or eczema, and a tendency to become easily overwhelmed when given too much information.

If your hypersensitivity is affecting your daily functioning, then you may have a sensory processing disorder (SPD). It is common for people living with ADHD to be diagnosed with SPD. In fact, according to studies, roughly 40 to 84% of patients living with ADHD also suffer from this disorder (Green, 2018). Unlike HSP, sensory processing disorder is a neurological condition that causes the brain to incorrectly process external information such as sound and light. This incorrect processing leads to overstimulation, stress, and other physiological symptoms. For example, sensitivity to light exposure could lead to painful photophobia.

Once again, a closer inspection of the sensory processing disorder can demonstrate to us how the mind-body connection works. SPD interrupts how the brain (the top of the central nervous system) organizes and interprets the messages that it receives through the body's receptors (through the eyes, ears, muscles, skin, etc.). This interruption means that internal sensory processing can falter, causing signals to misfire, and trouble in bodily movement, emotional experiences, and relationships with others can manifest.

One of the best ways to cope with sensory processing disorder is to become aware of the many ways it can manifest in your life. Below are examples of SPD symptoms at home and at work.

SPD Symptoms at Home

- You prefer to wear loose-fitting and light clothing that won't rub on your skin.
- During thunderstorms, you try to sleep or block out the sound because of the noise and appearance of lightning.
- While you enjoy the pool, being on the beach or swimming in a lake may feel uncomfortable when sand or mud brushes on your feet.
- Even though you adore your romantic partner, you would prefer it if they didn't give you big and tight hugs all the time.
- You find the bright flashes of a camera very uncomfortable.
- You find yourself becoming nauseous at the smell of certain perfumes, foods, and aromas.

- You find the taste of coffee too bitter.
- Sometimes, the texture of food can put you off a meal completely.

SPD Symptoms at Work

- When your colleague listens to music on their headphones, you find yourself wanting to ask them if they can turn it down.
- You would rather go hungry than eat food from the cafeteria that is mushy in texture.
- You always dread giving presentations due to a fear of stumbling on the words or getting distracted by the sound of coworkers whispering about something.
- The strong fluorescent light bulbs at work sometimes make you feel nauseous.
- You are not a fan of using Post-It notes because you can't read your own handwriting.
- Being in a cramped elevator with more than four people can make you hyperventilate and want to get off quickly.

Natural Remedies for Treating Sensory Processing Disorder

Having sensory processing disorder does not mean that you have to settle for a subpar life or accept that you will never enjoy many of the sensory experiences that most people find pleasurable. Treatment for this disorder usually includes therapies such as sensory integration therapy and occupational therapy. However, there are also smart home remedies you can try that have also been proven to be effective. Some of these natural home remedies are listed below.

1. Homeopathy

Some incredible homeopathic remedies have become popular over the years for their effectiveness in treating sensory processing disorder. Some of these include belladonna and Stramonium. When using homeopathic treatments, it is advised to speak to a professional who can guide you in taking the medicine correctly. This is especially important when taking such potent substances that are meant to alter your neurological functioning.

2. Cognitive Practice

If you have been diagnosed with sensory processing disorder, it is important that you engage in daily exercises to improve your cognitive function. These exercises will allow you to form new neural pathways to help you experience a more fulfilling life by, for instance, practicing self-awareness, interacting with others, and gradually exposing yourself to new experiences and sensations.

3. Salt Therapy

There have been numerous studies showing evidence that salt baths can be effective in treating certain hyperactive conditions and neurological disorders. An Epsom bath is one form of salt therapy that has been hailed for its health benefits for hundreds of years. You can simply pour the salt in your bath water and soak in it for at least 15 minutes, or you can prepare a foot bath by pouring Epsom salt in a small bucket of water. The salt bath is believed to have positive effects on those with sensory processing disorder by calming the nervous system, reducing their levels of anxiety, and promoting restful and deep sleep.

4. Altering Your Diet

Certain dietary foods can negatively impact neurological functioning and processes. Something as simple as paying careful attention to your diet may improve some of the symptoms that appear with this disorder. For instance, many people have found that removing all grains from their diet is helpful in regulating the body and preventing gastrointestinal issues. One of the diets that promotes this kind of lifestyle is the Paleo diet. However, it is important to speak to a nutritionist or trained specialist before committing to the diet.

5. Skullcap

Skullcap is one of the most popular and powerful herbs available on the market to treat sensory processing disorder. It contains strong nervine properties that can improve cognitive function and strengthen the connections of the brain. This can also help to prevent the onset of neurological disorders and is especially useful when treating sensory-based motor disorders.

6. Ginseng

Ginseng has been used as a remedy in China for several hundred years. It can improve cognition, increase your levels of concentration, and enhance the proper function of neurotransmitters. It can be consumed as an over-the-counter supplement or ingested in other forms. You can peel the raw ginseng root and chew on it or cut the raw root into slices and boil it in water to make tea.

7. Melatonin Boost

There has been research conducted that links low levels of melatonin with sensory processing disorder. Melatonin is a hormone released by the pea-sized pineal gland located just above the middle of your brain. This hormone is what tells your body to go to sleep and wake up. Low levels of melatonin can lead to insomnia, mental fatigue, and physical exhaustion, some of the typical symptoms that accompany SPD. You can invest in natural melatonin supplements, reduce artificial lights at night, reduce your levels of stress, and incorporate melatonin-rich foods like pineapples, bananas, oranges, tomatoes, and sweet corn in your diet.

ADHD and Rejection Sensitive Dysphoria

At some point in our lives, most of us will be concerned about what others think of us. This is normal, especially when we find ourselves in social settings or intimate relationships with others. This natural concern about the message we are conveying to others or how they perceive us opens us up to experiencing rejection.

Regardless of who you are and where you come from, rejection affects you the same way it affects me—it's painful. Social rejection in particular activates the same parts of the brain that physical pain does, and the experience of social rejection and physical pain have many similarities on a brain scan. Nevertheless, some of us are more sensitive to rejection than others or perceive that we are being rejected in many situations where we are not. In these cases, it is possible to experience what is known as rejection sensitive dysphoria (RSD).

This condition has only recently been discovered and more research aiming to understand it is currently underway. However, there are a few things we do know about RSD. People who have this condition tend to react negatively to the perception of being rejected. Their experience of rejection goes far beyond the normal feeling of distress, humiliation, or discomfort that someone may feel.

People who have RSD experience such a strong emotional reaction to criticism, exclusion, or judgment from others that it leads to mental, emotional, and, many times, physical side-effects. Even perceived judgment from someone else can completely ruin their day, making them feel like a failure and act in ways disproportionate to the exchange that actually occurred. It is common for those with RSD to exaggerate the exchange that takes place between themselves and others and believe that people are against them. This exaggerated response can lead to either rage or carrying a heavy feeling of shame. It may also cause some individuals to become people-pleasers, going above and beyond for others in a desperate attempt to make themselves lovable. Meanwhile, others may look at people with RSD and perceive them as being overly sensitive, perfectionists, or dramatic.

It is important to distinguish between RSD and social anxiety disorder. Social anxiety disorder is one of the most common psychological disorders in the United States. It involves the preoccupation and distress associated with the fear of being judged negatively by others. Most people who have social anxiety disorder experience it in social settings, from chatting to strangers in an elevator to having small talk at a party. Their discomfort in social settings is so prominent that they would rather avoid going out or interacting with others totally (or feel miserable when they force themselves or are forced to socialize).

Rejection sensitive dysphoria has some similarities to social anxiety disorder, and the two conditions can occur in the same person and feed off each other at times. However, RSD does differ from social anxiety disorder. For instance, someone who has RSD won't necessarily feel distressed when meeting new people or engaging in social interactions—their main issue is feeling rejection in those social settings. Moreover, a person with RSD won't feel anxious before a presentation or interaction with another person, but they will have an exaggerated emotional reaction afterward if they felt the engagement didn't go well. Therefore, instead of feeling nervous about social interactions like one who has social anxiety disorder would, the person with RSD is plagued with guilt, rage, and shame when they experience what they perceive to be rejection.

Adults with ADHD are at risk of experiencing RSD. This is because the central nervous system tends to be triggered differently in people who have ADHD. For instance, an adult with ADHD may sense signals that they are being perceived in a way that makes them the "other", thus creating a tumultuous cycle. Furthermore, the tendency to act impulsively, which is associated with ADHD, can make a person respond to social interactions in a way that sabotages relationships or causes misunderstandings.

RSD in adults living with ADHD can manifest in two ways. First, the emotional response can be directed inwardly. RSD can sometimes feel like a complete mood disorder such as depression, and if it isn't addressed within reasonable time, it may lead to suicidal thoughts. Other times, the quick transition from feeling fine to feeling immensely sad can lead to misdiagnosing RSD for bipolar disorder. Secondly, RSD can manifest as an emotional response directed outwardly. This may lead to outbursts of rage directed at the specific person or situation that has supposedly judged, criticized, or undermined the person with RSD. Living with RSD is exhausting because it can make people who are living with ADHD constantly expect rejection from others. Many times, this rejection is triggered by past emotional pain or by the perceived or real loss of love, respect, and approval.

Mentalizing as a Treatment for Rejection Sensitive Dysphoria

Mentalizing refers to the unforced sense we have of ourselves and others as people whose behaviors and actions are based on mental states. We understand that our actions are based on feelings, desires, beliefs, and unmet needs. Usually, when we are interacting with other people, we automatically go beyond face value, basing our response on what we perceive of the other person's behavior.

Therefore, we can say that all human beings are active mind readers, always attempting to understand people's true intentions and will. Mentalizing involves accurate mind-reading in order to understand the mind and actions of others without assuming that they are thinking or feeling the same way we are. Adopting this unbiased understanding of another person is not as easy to do as it sounds. This is because mental states are constantly fluctuating, and what someone intended yesterday may be different from what they do today. This also applies to your reasoning, beliefs, emotions, and thoughts. What you felt or thought a few years, months, or weeks ago has morphed into another feeling or thought.

The reason why learning how to mentalize is an important exercise in psychiatric treatment is that it helps you separate your mind from the other person's mind, thereby seeing the interaction with more sober eyes. For instance, someone who lives with rejection sensitive dysphoria may try to explain the actions of others through their own mental and emotional conclusions. Thus, what they perceive as rejection is immediately assumed to be true. However, if this individual took time to separate his or her mind and actions from that of the other person, they wouldn't be so quick to see the outcome of the situation as a form of rejection. Instead, they would put themselves in the other person's shoes and find that there may have been other underlying feelings, thoughts, and beliefs that could be responsible for how they acted or behaved.

Mentalizing is a valuable skill that you can use in interactions with all people, whether it is on a professional or personal level. This skill will always be necessary because you will meet different kinds of individuals with various mental and emotional motivations. Effective mentalizing will help you stay flexible and not be so offended by people who act in ways that are different from what you are used to. You will be able to understand, at the very least, that they have a reasonable explanation for why they behave in the manner they do.

One of the first things to understand about mentalizing is that it can be explicit or implicit. By this, I mean that mentalizing can be a conscious exercise that you are aware is taking place or a more intuitive exercise that you are not consciously aware of. When you mentalize consciously, you notice the strange actions or behaviors of others and consciously explore the possible reasons for their actions. You may ask yourself, "Why is this person treating me in this manner? Is he frustrated that I was unable to return his phone call earlier today?"

Another way to mentalize consciously is to actively explore the reasons behind your own behaviors (similar to the practice of self-awareness). For instance, you may ask yourself, "Why did I act so shy in front of those people? Was I self-conscious about what they would think about my ideas?" When you are preoccupied with making sense of your external and internal world, you are actively mentalizing.

However, thinking about your intentions and the intentions of others is only a part of mentalizing—there is also implicit mentalizing which is performed intuitively. A majority of the interactions you have with others is intuitive, meaning that you hardly think about what you are going to say or what the other person's response will be. It's the same as riding a bicycle; the first couple of times meeting someone, you are conscious of how you present yourself and what you say. However, as you get comfortable with them, your interactions become a habit.

Thus, while mentalizing can occur on an intellectual level, it can also take place on a gut level. Think about how you respond to another person's emotion of excitement or sadness. Since you have registered these emotions in your mind, chances are high that you will respond automatically with an emotion that matches the one that is being conveyed. Another example of implicit mentalizing is seen in how two people engaging in a dialogue will naturally take turns to speak. This is not something that they are conscious of but rather an automatic response to the situation.

Explicit and implicit mentalizing is part of the foundation of self-awareness and distinguishing your identity from others'. Mentalizing also gives you a sense of self-agency—being in complete control of your actions and behaviors and knowing what isn't sitting well with you at all times. Rejection, for instance, is a strong emotion that you may feel. It is also something that you may seek to get therapy for once you identify it to be a recurring reason behind your social anxiety or dysfunctional relationships with others.

Mentalizing can help you isolate what you feel from what others are feeling. This reduces the likelihood of you blaming other people for strong emotions that you feel about yourself. For example, the bursts of anger that you sometimes experience could be triggered by emotional pain within yourself and not necessarily what someone said or did. Thus, mentalizing can positively improve your mental health by giving you a sense of ownership and responsibility for your actions, behaviors, and decisions instead of citing them as symptoms of ADHD, thus making them factors that are out of your control.

Did you know that mentalizing can also strengthen your personal and professional relationships? When you understand that you are a unique individual who is living a unique life experience, you are able to accept others for their quirks, flaws, and uniqueness. Mentalizing will help you see that everybody has a different view of life that's informed by their own thoughts, beliefs, emotions, etc. This gives you a chance to learn from everyone you interact with instead of avoiding those who may see the world differently from you. It also gives others a chance to learn from your experiences and understand life through your eyes.

In this sense, social interactions become more about sharing who you are and allowing others the opportunity to do the same. From this viewpoint, it doesn't matter if you are different from others; in fact, it is expected that you will be different. Your objective isn't about fitting in or adopting other people's outlooks on life. Rather, your objective is to learn something new that you perhaps have never thought of before or feel emotions that you hardly feel.

By practicing putting yourself in another person's shoes and seeing life from their perspective, you can naturally increase your ability to empathize with others. However, doing so doesn't mean losing yourself in another person's world. While empathizing, you should still maintain self-awareness, checking in with yourself about what you are thinking and feeling and how your body is responding to what the other person is sharing.

This intuitive empathizing with yourself and others allows the relationships in your life to flourish without you feeling like you need to hide who you are or withdraw from uncomfortable interactions. You will be able to embrace different types of interactions and adjust the verbal and emotional signals you read in other people's behavior.

For instance, you may notice that your coworkers looked disinterested at the beginning of a presentation. However, as you adjust your presentation style and look each one in the eyes, they became less distracted and more engaged in what you are saying. Another example is during small talk at a social gathering. You may notice that, initially, the other person is excited to get to know you, but as the conversation progresses, they start to look around for their friends. At that moment, you decide to ask this person a string of meaningful questions that will encourage them to share parts of themselves that make them happy. Suddenly, the person's mood changes and they are more jovial again.

ADHD and Stress

Stress is a normal part of everyday life, and so is our response to it. The physiological response to stress—which is typically characterized by a fight-or-flight response—is our body's way of keeping us alive. So, what does a normal stress response look like? Well, first, your heart will begin racing, and you will perhaps experience sweaty palms, as well as a sharp increase of adrenaline and cortisol through your body, which helps to make you more focused and alert.

The stress response was designed to help us in crisis situations alone, occurring for only brief periods of time. When we experience stress in the right doses, it can actually help us perform better due to increased mental alertness and strength. We were never supposed to live under chronic stress, with cortisol flushing through our bodies constantly. This type of scenario would give us very little relief from the racing heartbeat, increase in blood pressure, and other effects on our health and functioning.

Chronic stress is the toxic kind of stress that is ongoing in nature. When the brain feels continually threatened by factors in the environment, it tends to shut down in a bid to protect itself from further injury. This doesn't mean that the brain stops working; it continues to function. However, it does so at a much slower rate, exposing the individual to undesirable mental conditions like anxiety, depression, and a decrease in resilience to overcoming stress.

Adults with ADHD are more susceptible to experiencing toxic stress due to the overwhelming reality of having to cope with mental and emotional impairments that make even the most simple exercise stressful. Due to constantly feeling anxious or ill-equipped to face the world, they tend to have a much greater sensitivity to anything stressful in their environment and a more intense and prolonged stress response. Moreover, this chronic stress may aggravate the common symptoms of ADHD, including symptoms like memory loss and other cognitive and emotional conditions.

There has been a great deal of research exploring the link between ADHD and the stress response. According to the American Institute of Stress, a majority of adults with ADHD report feeling stressed in many areas of their lives, with 73% of them experiencing psychological symptoms and 77% experiencing physiological symptoms. Researchers have also repeatedly found that ADHD symptoms are, to some degree, associated with stress, especially in adults who have inattentive ADHD.

Chronic stress makes ADHD symptoms worse, and in extreme cases, it can cause chemical changes in the brain, affecting daily functioning. The more stress someone experiences, the greater the reduction in the executive functioning abilities of the brain, leading to challenges with organizing information and managing strong emotions. In general, adults with ADHD who also have high levels of stress can experience a severe decline in cognitive self-regulation, impacting their cognitive abilities to make decisions, problem-solve, and set goals.

The Art of Managing ADHD-Related Stress

Even though stress is overwhelming when you have ADHD, it is manageable. This should be good news because it means that it is possible to live a life where you are not constantly anxious or feeling hopeless by stressful triggers. If you are living with ADHD, you may find it difficult to filter out excess stimuli from your attention. Being overly stimulated may create challenges when you are trying to focus on tasks and other responsibilities, and this heightens stress in everyday life situations.

Recognizing the stress that you are exposed to as a result of living with ADHD is the first step in managing its effects on your life. For instance, you may have an anxiety attack and believe that you are falling behind in your work, but meanwhile, it is the ADHD-related stress magnifying your symptoms.

It is, therefore, important to practice self-awareness when triggered by a stressful situation. Stop blaming yourself for experiencing the stress or anxiety and, instead, observe what the fear brought along by the stress is trying to say to you, show it loving attention, and gently release it. Below are some of the other ways to manage and overcome stress on an ongoing basis.

1. **Write It Down**

So much of the party happens inside your head, but how much of it do you express on paper? Journaling your thoughts and emotions has been proven to reduce stress. It's a healthy way to express your frustrations or jot down all of the small details you want to remember later. Writing down your thoughts and emotions also allows you to identify patterns of behavior that may be destructive. For instance, if you notice that whenever you do a certain task you feel miserable, you can look deeper into that task and find out what about it is causing resistance. Thus, with written evidence, you are more equipped to acknowledge and address some of your stressors.

2. Create a Schedule

A common feeling when you are stressed is not feeling in control. This feeling in itself is terrifying. Simple tasks like going to the grocery store may feel too daunting for you to manage. Creating a schedule allows you to plan tasks ahead of time, giving you more control over how you spend your time. In this way, when a task is approaching, you are already prepared to face it. You can also map your day, adding in breaks in between tasks and giving yourself much-needed time for self-care. Included in your schedule could be an agenda of what the task will involve, all of the requirements, and the things you need to prepare in advance.

3. Prioritize Your Physical Health

Prioritizing your physical health can reduce ADHD-related stress. In fact, regular exercise is so effective that it has been shown to be one of the best alternative treatments for ADHD. This is because physical exercise increases your levels of serotonin to help you fight against the effects that come as a result of chronic stress and the overproduction of cortisol. Exercise can also make you more resilient to stress, thereby increasing your stress threshold over time. Something as simple as taking a walk every day will significantly improve the health of your mind and body.

4. Maintaining a Healthy Diet

Certain foods such as tea, blueberries, and leafy greens have been proven to reduce stress levels and alleviate the symptoms associated with ADHD. However, consuming these healthy foods isn't enough; it is important for you to adopt a healthy diet. Carefully monitoring what you eat can regulate your blood sugar, reduce any tension, and help fight against other stressors in your body. Avoid consuming processed or sugary foods that can aggravate ADHD symptoms.

5. Always See the Glass As Half Full

Maintaining a positive outlook can reduce ADHD-related stress and the effects of other stressors in your professional or personal life. Even when you feel like the stress is weighing you down, choose to see the positive aspects of the situation. I know that this isn't always easy to do, especially once you have been triggered. However, taking a few deep breaths and putting your mind in the present moment will bring you instant relief.

If you are stressed about your manager and how they are treating you, take a moment for yourself and practice a breathing exercise. Turn the situation around by thinking about all of the positive aspects of your job and what you are most grateful for. Use mentalizing to separate your mind and emotions from your manager's mind and emotions, and empathize with what they may be struggling with that would cause them to behave in the manner they are.

Reader Task: Breathing and Body Relaxation Exercise

Begin this exercise by finding a comfortable position to sit and rest your body. This may be on the floor or a chair. Feel free to close your eyes now, or if you are more comfortable keeping your eyes open, stare at a fixed focal point throughout the exercise.

Begin grounding your awareness into your body, feeling the weight of your body, the contact of your feet with the floor, and the contact of your back against the chair. Notice the parts of your body that are finding it difficult to remain still. Send those parts loving attention, and then bring your awareness back to your whole body. Once you feel that you are physically grounded, slowly bring your attention to your breath. Notice the natural pace of your breath, the sensation of your lungs expanding and contracting, and your natural pattern of breathing—inhalation, pause, exhalation.

If you notice that you are breathing from your chest, slow your breathing down and inhale deeper, with your breaths coming from your diaphragm. Enjoy the process of going deeper and deeper in your core with each round of breathing. The aim of this exercise is to slow down your breath until you reach a soothing pace that calms your mind and body.

During the exercise, you can follow a counting technique to time your breaths and slow your breathing gradually. The counting technique goes as follows:

Inhale for 4 counts, pause for 4 counts, and exhale for 4 counts.

Repeat the counting technique for a few rotations or until you are naturally following the rhythm. It is common to experience distractions while performing this exercise. When distractions do arise, identify them as simply passing thoughts, and bring your attention back to the counting technique:

Inhale for 4 counts, pause for 4 counts, and exhale for 4 counts.

Continue for as long as you need to. When you are feeling calm, begin the process of reorienting yourself with your surroundings. Bring your awareness to your body; slowly start moving your toes, fingers, shoulders, and so on until your full body is awake. Prepare for the next task or activity in your day. Remember that you can repeat this exercise at any other point in the day when you feel overwhelmed, stressed, or tense.

Chapter 5:

Thinking Your Way to Health

Negative thinking can become a spiral that we all get caught up in sometimes. However, when it becomes habitual, it can cause devastating impacts on our overall well-being and mental health. Science has continuously shown how positive thinking can actually have the opposite effect. Thinking positively about our lives can improve our general well-being and mental health.

So, what can be considered negative thinking? If you are a person who is prone to overthinking and analyzing your own thoughts, you may find it difficult to spot when you are in a cycle of negative thinking or when you are carrying the same concerns that everyone else has. For instance, being worried that you are going to miss an appointment, stressing over your financial burdens, or having concerns about your relationships is absolutely normal. The issue only comes when these thoughts occur frequently, repetitively, and intrusively.

If I had to define negative thinking, I would describe it as adopting an innately negative belief system about yourself and others that consequently affects your daily functioning, work, future aspirations, and relationships. This thought pattern builds mental blocks that inhibit you from seeking help, forming strong connections with others, having plans for your future, or practicing self-awareness. I have frequently heard people describe negative thinking as being locked up in the prison of your own mind, unable to set yourself free or let others close to you. As a result of this withdrawal from actively participating in your life or connecting with others, there comes a strong sense of separation, depression, and anxiety.

It is important to note that not everyone who thinks negatively has a mental illness, and not everyone with a mental illness thinks negatively. However, negative thinking can sometimes be influenced by conditions such as obsessive compulsive disorder (OCD), generalized anxiety disorder (GAD), and mental illnesses. Negative thinking may also be caused by three factors, which are outlined below.

1. Fear of the Future

It is common for many people to fear the unknown and how their future will pan out. The fear of the future tends to lead to catastrophizing, which is the habit of predicting the worst-case scenario or future failures when thinking about what is to come. The only way to effectively deal with this fear is to transport your mind to the present moment and realize that the only time that you can influence is the here and now.

2.   Anxiety About the Present

It is understandable to be anxious about the present and how you will cope with the issues that you are currently facing. You may also be worried about what others think of you, whether you are suited for your job, how your ADHD symptoms will flare up, or how the traffic will be on your way home. People who are negative thinkers create worse case scenarios for present challenges. For example, they may believe that no one really likes them at work, they are on the brink of getting fired, or they won't be able to cope with stress.

The fear of the present moment is usually linked to the fear of losing control. However, when people realize that there are many factors that are not under their control, they can lift some of the weight from their shoulders.

3.   Shame About the Past

Carrying shame about the past can keep you lying awake at night unable to sleep. It is a toxic tormenting feeling of regret and a string of thoughts about how you could have done things better. The truth is that everyone has done and said things that they are embarrassed about when they think back about them. Who you were a few years ago is completely different from who you are now.

Negative thinkers, however, cannot let the past go. They spend their days thinking obsessively about their childhood, adolescent years, past mistakes and failures, the death of loved ones, dreams that were never fulfilled, and so on. The only way to heal this feeling of shame is to accept the parts of your past that carry strong emotional pain. You can do this by seeking therapy and actively opening the doors of your past that you have kept shut for so long.

You don't have to settle for a life of negative thinking. There are many techniques that you can learn which will help you intercept negative thoughts before they consume your being. One technique is to practice countering exercises every time you have a negative thought and to avoid giving up or feeling disappointed when you slip up.

Below are five questions that you can ask yourself every time you have a negative thought. You can either answer these questions in your head or write them down in a journal.

1. Is this thought that I am having true? Is there a reasonable justification for this negative belief?
2. Is this thought giving me power, or is it taking my power away?
3. Is it possible for me to put a positive spin on this thought or learn something from it?
4. What would my life look like if I didn't have these negative beliefs?
5. Is this thought glossing over an issue that I need to address?

Self-Defeating Beliefs

Your belief system is made up of your attitudes, personal views, and values. This system is built within you, meaning that all of your behaviors and actions will be based on your beliefs and that it is impossible for you to escape from them. Your beliefs shape the way you see yourself and the world around you. They display your level of commitment, ambition, resilience, and optimism about your life, work, and relationships.

Empowering beliefs can positively transform your life, giving you the strength and conviction to achieve outstanding goals that you set for yourself. Self-defeating beliefs, on the other hand, will slowly cause you to cave in to your own life and stunt your personal development. It is ironic that people who have self-defeating beliefs fear failure the most. Carrying these negative beliefs sets you up for failure and promotes a life of fear.

Self-defeating beliefs fall into two categories, namely intrapersonal and interpersonal negative beliefs. So, what's the difference? Intrapersonal self-defeating beliefs are negative beliefs projected externally. Someone with these may be a perfectionist at work, seek approval from their peers, or believe that their sense of self-worth is determined by their external achievements. Conversely, those who have interpersonal self-defeating beliefs carry negative beliefs that are experienced on a personal level. For instance, they may blame themselves for the mistakes of others, become submissive to a fault, or fear getting involved in conflict.

These self-defeating beliefs (whether intrapersonal or interpersonal) create negative thinking patterns. Negative thinking patterns are not so easy to identify because they will only appear when someone is faced with an issue. For example, when you are presented with a crisis, negative thoughts will come rushing to your mind, and these thoughts will reinforce your self-defeating beliefs.

If you are a person who finds your sense of self-worth in your achievements, it will be difficult for you to identify a negative thinking pattern when everything is going well and you are accomplishing your goals. However, as soon as you face an obstacle, your negative thinking pattern may be activated, leading you to start over-analyzing your actions, questioning your own abilities, and dealing with negative self-talk which then triggers anxiety.

Your negative thoughts may make you think that you are a failure and that you are to blame for how the situation has transpired. You may say to yourself, "Clearly, this wasn't meant to be," or, "I'll never be able to make it." Over time, these habitual negative thoughts may lead to low self-esteem, chronic stress, and depression. Personal beliefs are learned over time through how you have handled various life experiences. Because they have been so ingrained in your lifestyle, it is difficult to change how you think, feel, and interpret the world overnight.

Nevertheless, there are ways to break the cycle of self-defeating beliefs and negative thought patterns for good. The best place to start is learning to recognize where and when self-defeating beliefs appear in your life. They may be concentrated in a particular area of your life that you feel insecure or have deep unresolved emotional pain about. Start noticing your outlook on life, your thoughts on various aspects of who you are, and how you respond to different problems.

For instance, there may be problems that you can easily rectify or cope with and others that just make you go into a panic and freeze up. It is also important to recognize how you deal with issues. Are you the type of person who faces problems head-on, or do you succumb to negative thoughts that paralyze you, preventing you from taking any action?

As soon as you identify a self-defeating belief or negative thinking pattern, face it. Question the validity of these thoughts and try to figure out where they could have come from. Dispute and dispose of these beliefs, in turn replacing them with ones that are more authentic to who you are and what you are capable of doing. Instead of believing that you are an embarrassment for failing at a task, you may find that you are just really disappointed that you couldn't follow through with the plan, but also accept that you are growing and learning from every setback.

Automatic Negative Thinking

When you physically hurt yourself and develop a cut on your skin, the treatment is straightforward: you can rinse the affected area with water, apply antibacterial cream, and wrap the wound with a bandage. After some time, the cut will heal and you will remove the bandage, continuing with life as normal.

Treating years of negative thinking takes on a more complicated nature, especially when your thoughts stem from chronic anxiety, depression, or any other mental health condition. Treatment for negative thinking may be different for each individual. It can require different approaches to psychotherapy and various lifestyle changes. However, you can also treat yourself at home by making mental shifts. Mental shifts refer to the process of consciously changing the way you think about yourself and your life, bringing an end to an established thought pattern or habit. It involves reevaluating how you look at various situations and the response you have toward them. It's like shifting mental gears so that your thought processes are not constantly reinforcing negative beliefs.

By making mental shifts, you will, in essence, undo all of the negative belief systems and programming you have been controlled by for so many years. For example, if you grew up with the pressure to perform at the top of your class at school, you may be programmed to be a perfectionist, causing you a lot of stress and anxiety in life. A mental shift would pull you out of this loop and allow you to determine new perspectives and beliefs regarding your performance and capabilities.

Why "Should" Is a Toxic Word

If you notice that your thoughts include "should" a lot, take a pause. Statements with the word "should" involved could contribute to anxious thought patterns because they place an expectation on you that may, at times, be impossible for you to accomplish. Examples of "should" statements include:

- "I should think, act, or feel better."
- "I should go to the gym 5 times per week."
- "I should change my diet and eat healthier foods."
- "I should stop procrastinating."

Don't get me wrong—the intention behind these statements may be good. Depending on your lifestyle, it might be beneficial for you to eat better. However, the problem with these "should" statements is that they set the bar so high that they can trigger guilt, frustration, and self-defeating beliefs. Imagine the spiral that would take place if three weeks pass and you are still procrastinating or you haven't been able to be consistent with going to the gym.

Very few people will tell you this, but the path toward mental, emotional, and physical freedom can be messy. By messy I mean that you will make mistakes and your journey won't be as clear-cut as you expect it to be. As I have mentioned, most of these negative thought patterns are ingrained, and it takes more than a few attempts to completely break the cycle. Therefore, instead of telling yourself that you should do something, intercept the thought with more empowering thoughts like these:

- "I will try my best to catch myself thinking negatively or when I'm triggered by strong emotions by doing the following…"
- "When I am unable to go to the gym, I can still improve my health by doing the following…"
- "I can eat healthier this week by taking these simple actions…"
- "I notice that I am procrastinating right now. What's a better way to spend my time? What advice would I give a friend who was in the same situation?"

Behind every "should" statement may be a form of cognitive distortion that is known as automatic negative thinking (ANT) or having automatic negative thoughts. Automatic negative thoughts are usually the first thoughts you have when you experience a strong feeling or reaction to something. These are relentless and have been learned through many years of mental programming. They are often reiterating themes such as danger or fear and are more prevalent in people living with anxiety or depression. Therefore, recognizing automatic negative thinking when you live with a mental health condition may be extremely difficult.

One of the ways to identify and overcome automatic negative thinking is by keeping a thought record. In the previous chapter, I told you that journaling is very effective when dealing with stress because it allows you to see the nature and patterns of your thoughts. Journaling is also an effective technique to use for identifying subtle negative thoughts that have gone undetected for years.

In your thought record or journal, you would write about a triggering scenario that recently took place, breaking the scenario into three parts: the situation, your mood, and the thought or image that automatically sprung to mind. After having identified these three parts, you can go deeper with each one by asking yourself the following questions:

Part 1: What situation is causing your anxiety?

- Where were you?
- Who were you with at the time?
- What were you doing?
- When was it?

Part 2: What is your mood about this situation?

Describe the feelings that you felt in keywords, and then rate the intensity of these emotions on a percentage scale that totals 100%. The aim of rating your feelings is to see how much of your thoughts were influenced by a particular emotion. You might record your moods like this:

- Irritated = 15%

- Disrespected = 10%
- Rejected = 50%
- Insecure = 25%

Part 3: What are the automatic negative thoughts racing through your mind?

Part 3 is the most important step in your thought record. This is because the answers you get from it will direct you to some of the self-defeating beliefs you carry within you. You can simply list the thoughts, images, or ideas that came through your mind at the time. Some of these automatic negative thoughts may include:

- "I'm so dumb."
- "I'll never be better than..."
- "I know I'm going to embarrass myself again."
- "I always disappoint myself."
- "Everyone pretends to like me."
- "I am a burden on others."
- "Life is unfair."
- "I'm not supposed to be here."
- "I can't cope with this."
- "I'm going to end up alone."

If you find yourself always caught up in these automatic negative thoughts or ones like them, the act of breaking down the triggering scenario will help you isolate your thoughts from what actually happened and how the situation made you feel. Without breaking the scenario down, it can be easy for you to forget about the various factors that led up to the negative thought, which probably have a lot more to do with your mood than you realize.

For instance, if your automatic negative thought is "I know I'm going to embarrass myself again", you can look to the situation for more answers as to why you have been triggered in this way. If it's a work-related situation, ask yourself whether you are fearful of being rejected due to past projects that didn't go so well. Now, think of all the ways that this current situation is actually different from past projects. Break down your moods and feelings to see if this automatic negative thought is valid or just a symptom of fear. Now, think of ways you can change the script and replace your negative thought with a more empowering thought like "I will do the best that I can with the knowledge that I have".

The Link Between Positive Thinking and Mental Health

It's true—positive thinking can help you manage stress and improve your mental well-being. I always ask people this simple question: Is your glass half empty or half full? It can reveal to me the outlook you carry about your life and the attitude you have about yourself. People who tend to see the glass as half empty are known to be pessimistic and those who choose to see the glass as half full are optimists. Personality traits like being optimistic or being pessimistic can affect your mental health. Optimists prefer to see the world in a positive way, and this may reduce their levels of stress in daily functioning.

Positive thinking has been misunderstood over the years and painted as a very ignorant and "head in the sand" type of approach to dealing with challenging situations and living a fulfilling life. At its core, positive thinking is simply the choice to face unpleasant circumstances in a more productive and encouraging way. Instead of thinking that the worst is going to happen, you decide to think that you will survive and continue to thrive despite the outcome.

Positive thinking always starts with how you speak to yourself about yourself. This is also referred to as self-talk. Self-talk is the endless stream of thoughts that race through your head, many of which are never spoken to anybody else. These automatic thoughts can either be positive or negative, depending on your particular belief system. If you have become accustomed to negative self-talk, then there is a high chance that you have a pessimistic view of yourself and others. If your self-talk is mostly positive, then you are probably a very optimistic person.

Positive self-talk fueled by positive thinking has been known to promote the following health benefits:

- An increased life span
- Lower levels of depression
- Lower levels of stress
- A greater resistance to illnesses like the flu
- Healthier psychological and physiological well-being
- Better cardiovascular health
- A greater resilience and better coping skills when hit with hard times

There are many people who would love to adopt positive thinking, but they are unclear about what positive and negative self-talk looks like. If you are not sure what negative self-talk is, you can read about some common instances that will cause you to go into a negative thought spiral below to gain a better understanding of the concept.

Filtering: If you are a person who highlights the negative aspects of a situation and downplays the positive ones, you may be guilty of filtering. For instance, you might have had a great day at work and completed your tasks on time, but when you get home, you are over-focused on the dishes that you forgot to wash, the dinner you still need to cook, and the mess waiting for you in the bathroom.

Personalizing: Someone who is personalizing blames themselves whenever bad things occur. For instance, an evening out with a group of your friends might get canceled, and you immediately assume that it was because no one wanted to be around you.

Catastrophizing: When catastrophizing, you immediately anticipate the worst-case scenario happening. A common example is sitting in terrible traffic in the morning and anticipating the entire day to be filled with disappointment.

Polarizing: Someone who is polarizing sees things as being either good or bad; in essence, they have a black and white approach to situations. These people don't believe there is a middle ground or that second-best exists. They might see themselves as either perfect or a failure and never as a work in progress.

Once you have identified negative thought patterns and negative self-talk, it becomes a lot easier to turn things around and begin to think more positively. It's worth mentioning, however, that the process takes time and constant practice. Be gentle with yourself as you reprogram your mind and begin to shift your mentality; you are creating a new habit, and this isn't an overnight process. Below are some ways to think and start behaving in a more positive way.

Identify areas that you would like to change: If you desire to think more positively about yourself and your life, you will need to identify areas of your life that you tend to think negatively about. This could include your job, personal relationships, mental health condition, or the commute to work. You can take baby steps by focusing on one area at a time.

Check in with yourself: Regularly throughout the day, pause for a minute and evaluate what you are thinking about. If you find that your thoughts are self-defeating, place a positive twist on them, and encourage yourself to see the glass as half full.

Embrace humor: Humor is truly the best form of medicine. It reminds us that we are all finding our own way in this crazy world, and that it doesn't have to look a certain way. Give yourself permission to smile and laugh. Find the humor in daily happenings, like how you left the keys in the door or how when you got to the grocery store, you had forgotten what you needed in the first place. Laughing at yourself reduces tension and stress and also helps you accept the life that you are leading.

Surround yourself with positive people: Ensure that the people closest to you are positive. While you may not be able to control how your colleagues behave, at least you can control who you go home to. Positivity is infectious; when one person can't help but have hope in their lives, it rubs off on those around them. Positive people can offer you support when you are feeling low and help you see all of the possibilities in your life. Negative people are already prone to stress, and this may cause them to project their own fears and insecurities onto you. Therefore, you should never compromise when it comes to the quality of people you keep close.

Practice positive self-talk: Positive self-talk promotes positive thinking. You can practice positive self-talk by learning to follow one simple rule: Don't think anything about yourself that you would never publicly say to anyone else. Would you call your friend dumb or tell them that they will never amount to anything? I'm sure you wouldn't. Positive self-talk requires you to set a standard of what you can and cannot say about yourself. Be gentle and compassionate with yourself, similarly to how you would be with a baby who is learning how to walk for the first time. The truth is that you are also learning to walk again by transforming how you see your life and the world around you.

Positive Affirmations for Healing

Every day, your body experiences physical changes in response to the quality of thoughts that continuously run through your mind. Just thinking about something small and insignificant causes your brain to send signals throughout your body and release neurotransmitters. Neurotransmitters control virtually all of your bodily functions, including your emotions. Over a number of years—and with repetition—your thoughts can change the architecture of your brain, cells, and even genes.

A good example is when people practice gratitude. The conscious awareness of the positive aspects of your life sends a surge of rewarding neurotransmitters like dopamine throughout your body. This ultimately causes you to feel more uplifted and positive about your life. Even science acknowledges that what you visualize, think about, and say to yourself can change your body, brain, and emotional well-being. One way to actively harness the power of your thoughts is through practicing reciting positive affirmations.

Affirmations are simply thoughts that you intentionally create to support, empower, and calm your mind and body. There have been studies showing that positive affirmations can help you respond in a less defensive way when you are presented with a stressful situation. These positive statements are used as weapons to counter negative and anxiety-producing thoughts and beliefs.

Over time, affirmations are effective tools that you can utilize to break free from negative thinking patterns, habits, and moods. Here are some of the proven benefits of positive affirmations:

- Reduced stress levels
- Better coping with threatening situations with less resistance
- Boosted academic or professional achievements
- Increased feeling of hopefulness about the future
- Improved self-esteem and confidence

You can use affirmations in any life situation where you would like to see positive change take place. For instance, you may want to recite affirmations before going into a meeting, when feelings of anxiety arise, when you need to find the motivation to continue with a task, or when you wish to quit a self-defeating habit.

Affirmations are always more effective when they are practiced alongside other positive thinking techniques. For example, after writing your thought record and having successfully identified the automatic negative thought, you can recite a few affirmations that will remind you of the positive aspects of yourself and your capabilities.

Another example is practicing affirmations with a breathing technique. When you catch yourself engaging in a negative thought during the day, you can first take slow and relaxing breaths, and once you are calm, you can recite positive affirmations to yourself.

It is also important to note that your affirmations will be based on statements that are unique to you. You can think about your ideal state of mind, physical health, and emotional well-being and create affirmations that promote this higher version of yourself. You can also use affirmations that are based on the specific things you desire to achieve in your life, as well as the issues you seek to address.

Positive Affirmations to Help You Deal With Anxiety

If you are someone who battles with anxiety, it is important for you to halt anxiety-producing thoughts before they become all-consuming. Affirmations can assist you with that; you can recall positive beliefs about yourself whenever you need the extra boost of confidence or reassurance. Here are a few examples of positive affirmations that can help you reduce your anxiety and turn a situation around positively:

- "I am freeing myself from fear, judgment, and worry."
- "I choose to encourage myself with positive thoughts."
- "My anxiety does not control my life."
- "I can handle this task with ease."
- "I am safe."
- "This is not a crisis, and I don't need to panic ."
- "I will overcome this feeling."
- "I will figure out the next step naturally."
- "This situation is temporary."

Positive Affirmations to Help You Deal With Depression

Similarly to anxiety, depression can cause you to deal with a loop of negative thoughts and make you feel weak in comparison to the challenges that you face. Positive affirmations can help you transform your thinking patterns and general outlook on life by acknowledging and deliberately focusing on the positive aspects of yourself and your life. Here are a few examples of positive affirmations for overcoming depression:

- "I am valuable, even when I am not productive."
- "Despite my sadness, I am loved."
- "I am learning and growing to love myself every day."
- "My brain is my friend."
- "I am appreciated, even when I cannot contribute much."
- "I am needed."
- "I am separate from my depression."
- "I am more than the negative opinions I have of myself."
- "My discomfort won't last forever."
- "I am okay where I am right now."

You have the power to influence your mental and physical well-being with your thoughts. It is your responsibility to use this power to your advantage. While you cannot control what happened in the past—which shaped your brain, programmed your cells, and influenced your genes—you can choose the quality of thoughts that you have, and this will influence your behavior, record new information in your brain, and bring mental and physical rejuvenation.

Chapter 6:

ADHD Is Not the Enemy, Fear Is

Do you ever wish that you had somebody in your life who is always calm, cool, and collected—a voice of reason that you could turn to for clarity and a sense of order? Well, it turns out we're all built with something that provides us with this ability; it's known as the prefrontal cortex. However, for adults living with ADHD, the prefrontal cortex takes on a very different tone.

Instead of helping them focus and find the best solution in a crisis situation, it can cause fear and anxiety to take over, usually making the crisis feel worse than it already is. Since the calm, still voice of the prefrontal cortex is not activating the brain in the manner that it should, the mind of a person with ADHD is usually working overtime to compensate for their cognitive impairment. However, their emotional intelligence and empathy are diminished.

Many adults with ADHD become so overwhelmed by fear that they avoid it at all costs. Unfortunately, avoiding fear compromises one's quality of life. By staying away from everything that is a possible threat, your life becomes very small, and soon you find yourself afraid or reluctant to do activities or work that used to be a part of your daily life. Fear is a thief that comes to steal everything in your life—from your joy to your peace. It hides under a disguise, appearing to be something that can protect you from possible danger, but truth be told, it comes to delay you from being yourself and living an authentic life.

When you are triggered by fear, you will think back on traumatic past events or come up with the worst thoughts about your future. Soon enough, you will start making fear-based decisions about your life like not driving on a certain road, using only one form of transportation, visiting a specific place, or eating particular foods.

The reason why many people allow the voice of fear to torment them for so many years is that they believe these warnings or precautions are for their own good. They think that the more insulated they are from trouble, the happier they will be. The problem is that fear doesn't insulate us from trouble—it makes us afraid of it.

You have all of the resources within you to overcome every obstacle that you will ever face. This is because every barrier was, to some degree, created by your own mental, emotional, and physiological states. In other words, since the root of the obstacle is internal, you have all the tools required to reverse the signals, information, and programming that you have been living under. After realizing this truth about yourself, fear becomes an unnecessary exercise.

The voice of fear that is so audible in your ears receives its strength when you believe that the fake warning shots are true. So what is the best way to silence this voice? Assume that you don't know anything about your life and that you are waiting for the future to unfold for you. Fear is fueled by your need to be in control of what happens in your life, work, and relationships. This obsessive need to control factors in your environment ends up putting a lot of pressure on you.

Let's face it—there are some things that you will never fully understand or completely control. Even your ADHD symptoms are at best manageable and can improve over time, but they cannot be fully controlled. Your future prospects at work, the likelihood of you getting a promotion, and how others perceive you to be are simply things you cannot manipulate or influence as much as you try.

Fear seems to lose its grip when you realize and accept that you have no control over how things will play out, but your optimistic outlook on life keeps you hopeful. Your freedom from the shackles of fear lies in not knowing. Admitting that you don't know is not an admission of defeat, but rather it is an acceptance of your limited strength as a human being to control matters beyond your own comprehension. Anxiety, fear, and doubt cease to exist when you assume that you don't have all of the answers. This is because doubt comes about as a self-imposed obligation or expectation to have to know.

Fear also appears as a result of feeling a low sense of self-worth or that who you are and how you are living is wrong. This creates a deep feeling of guilt and the belief that you deserve to suffer. Ironically, people are more accepting of suffering than healing because of the hidden belief that suffering is a better form of correction and learning to be a better person. Suffering then becomes the fearful individual's teacher, placing the individual at its mercy, relentlessly repairing their personal image and constantly urging them to identify themselves with their pain.

Defense mechanisms become a tool to keep the person aligned with their suffering and prevent them from opening their heart, releasing emotional pain, and healing. At times, the attack is also directed at oneself by silencing every attempt to speak up and express how one truly feels, thinks, or desires. This is known as self-punishment, a cruel strategy to protect old narratives of pain and block the individual from breaking free of negative habits and patterns.

It's not that being fearful is wrong. I don't believe that there is a single person living on this earth who has never or will never experience fear. As we face new life experiences or outgrow older versions of ourselves, we will be struck by fear. However, the question is not whether you are fearful, but what you do with the fear once you recognize it. There are some who will decide to stand tall and courageously despite fearful situations and those who will shake at the knees and freeze. The boldness of the former gives them the opportunity to play out the full experience and learn from the outcome. The resistance of the latter robs them of the opportunity to build immunity to that kind of stressful experience and, thus, they will always be controlled by this particular circumstance.

When you have two options presented to you, one being more fearful than the other, and you choose the one you are less fearful of, you did not make the choice —your fear did. However, if instead you chose the option that frightened you the most, it might seem like a form of self-sabotage, but in actuality, it isn't. You are putting to shame the parts of you that hold you back from gathering as many life experiences as possible— the parts of you that worry what other people think or that feel embarrassed about you being authentically yourself.

At the end of the day, there is only one decision that you will have to make time and time again: Whether you will trust or fear. Choosing to trust means deciding to surrender to your life, who you are, and how your journey is progressing. On the other hand, choosing fear is deciding to fight for control and the survival of your ego. Seeking answers is also a way of fighting, and so is making judgments and comparisons. Therefore, the only obvious choice to make is trusting that your life will naturally unfold for you and that the outcome will be good.

Below are some strategies for preventing fear from controlling your life.

1. **Acknowledge that you are fearful.**

The first step to overcoming fear is to acknowledge that you are fearful. Coming to recognize this may be difficult, especially if you are someone who is uncomfortable with feeling fear. Nonetheless, the only way for it to stop claiming power over you is for you to call it out for what it is—a liar. Once you feel the fear in your belly or rising up to your chest, notice all of the emotions it has shut you off from feeling. Notice how your happiness, peace of mind, and positivity have disappeared. You can also notice what your fear is signaling as a possible threat or danger. Perhaps it is a boardroom meeting full of coworkers, a family gathering, or a night out on the town. Question whether the supposed threat is truly dangerous or just a poor attempt to make you shrink, lose confidence, and miss an opportunity.

2. Keep a list of effective coping strategies around.

It is always useful to have a list of coping strategies on hand in the event of a fearful thought suddenly coming to your mind and seeking to paralyze you. You can make this list on your phone, laptop, or on a piece of paper you carry around with you throughout the week. Planning coping strategies ahead of time gives you a chance to prepare and plan for how you will respond in fearful situations (where you are less likely to think on your feet about a quick solution). You can use new coping strategies and techniques that you have learned through your own research or stick to ones that have worked for you in the past.

3. Acknowledge that you are not perfect.

Seeking perfection can get in the way of living a fulfilling life. The desire to come out on top all of the time, succeed on your first try, and push yourself beyond reasonable limits will only bring fear and disappointment. When you set such a high standard for your life that causes you to put yourself on a pedestal, the pressure to maintain this persona or level of achievement will make you fear failure. When you acknowledge that you are not perfect and understand how to learn from your mistakes, fear can no longer accuse you of being worthless, lazy, or a disappointment to others. This gives you the space to continue pursuing your goals without having a constant standard to uphold.

4. Take each day as it comes.

Instead of telling yourself that you need to make it through the year, tell yourself that you need to get through each day. Narrowing your focus to a single day will reduce the anxiety that usually comes when we preoccupy ourselves with the future. It allows us to think of all the wonderful things that we would like to do each day and make it our mission to go ahead with them. It also means that we can face troubles one day at a time instead of thinking about how the crisis will unfold over several months or years. Reminding ourselves several times that we can make it through the day is all the encouragement we truly need.

Cultivating Happiness

We all desire to be happy, but sometimes our lives are full of so many stressors that this doesn't seem possible. Moreover, when we think of what happiness means to us, we may be likely to name external desires that our society teaches us to chase, such as making more money, being successful in our careers, improving our body image, or finding the perfect romantic lover. But are these genuinely our heart's desires? Research tends to think not, at least when it comes to long-term happiness. Losing weight, finding love, purchasing a home, or being recognized at work can give us a temporary feeling of happiness. Since human beings are naturally created to adapt to all circumstances, a new house will only feel new for the first few months or year; thereafter, it won't give you the same feeling of satisfaction as it did when you first got the keys.

Researchers in the field of psychology have found that it is possible to gradually increase your happiness with life, and it doesn't involve winning the lottery or having a dramatic life circumstance take place. Rather, it takes an inner adjustment of attitude and perspective. This implies that anybody can become happy and maintain happiness.

There are, however, many myths about happiness that cause people to feel stressed about their hopes for living a satisfying life. At times, these myths can cause many people to fear or feel undeserving of happiness due to what achieving happiness supposedly entails. Below are some of the myths that are simply not true about what happiness is and the ways to achieve it.

Myth: Money will make you happy.

You do need money to cover your basic survival needs, such as food, clothing, and a proper shelter. However, once you have enough money to live comfortably, acquiring more money won't make you any happier. Happiness is what causes you to enjoy your money and spend it on worthy pursuits. Thus, your happiness is more valuable than any currency in the world.

Myth: You need a relationship to be happy.

Your happiness is not tied to a romantic partner. Moreover, being single doesn't mean that you are unhappy or unfulfilled in some way. A relationship magnifies what you already are and allows your innermost emotions to show. Therefore, when an unhappy person enters a relationship, they quickly corrupt the union with their own toxic emotional baggage that they still need to deal with. Happy people always make good lovers because their self-awareness and true acceptance of who they are allows for the union to flourish and for both happy individuals to feed off each other's peace, joy, and compassion.

Myth: Happiness declines with age.

Contrary to what many believe, people tend to become happier as they get older. Studies have shown that seniors experience more positive and fewer negative emotions than younger people and middle-aged adults. Generally, the older one becomes, the more they reach the acceptance of life, thus feeling more satisfied with their lives and less stressed. Even with the losses that do come with age, older people are more emotionally stable to face challenges and enjoy what the present moment has to offer.

It may sound strange, but there is a formula for becoming happier about who you are and where you are in life. This formula is a combination of strategies that will enhance the quality of your life within hours of practicing them. Once again, practice makes perfect, and if you desire to turn these strategies into habits, then you will need to consciously practice performing them in your daily life as frequently as possible. Below are the various strategies for living a happier and more fulfilling life.

Strategy 1: Train your brain to think more positively.

The brain is wired in such a way that it remembers and records things that are wrong. This is a survival mechanism that helped keep our primitive ancestors safe in a world where there were many physical threats. In the present day, this biological predisposition has led to us naturally gravitating toward what's going wrong in our lives or goals that we still need to accomplish.

While we cannot change the nature of our brains, we *can* influence it to think positively. There are many ways of going about this, but one of the most powerful is to teach yourself to become more grateful. Expressing gratitude can reduce stress and anxiety in your life and cause you to become a happier person. You can express it through offering someone a simple thank you, keeping a gratitude journal and acknowledging five things each day that you are grateful for, or making it a habit to count your blessings and notice the small luxuries and comforts that have made your life more fulfilling.

Strategy 2: Nurture and enjoy your relationships.

Relationships are the greatest source of joy in our lives. Studies have shown that the happier the individual is, the more likely they are to have a supportive group of friends, a more fulfilling marriage, and a flourishing social life. This is why nurturing your relationships is one of the best emotional investments that you can make. As you become happier, you will attract happier people, too, and you will cultivate relationships that are based on mutual respect and acceptance.

Make it your priority to reach out to at least one person per week who you deem a close friend or relative. If you can, plan on going out for a quick coffee to catch up on what has been happening in your friends' lives, and, when appropriate, offer support and compliments to show that you truly value them. If you don't have any friends, this is a great opportunity to start seeking out happy people. When you are out running errands, shopping, or spending time on a hobby, strike a conversation with a few people and naturally invest more time getting to know those who have a contagiously positive personality.

Strategy 3: Live in the moment and appreciate every day.

When your mind is always focused on what is happening here or what you can do to make this moment better, you will always find happiness close by. You are more likely to notice the positive progress that is happening in the moment and feel more grateful than if you were to think back on the past or focus on the future.

One of the exercises you can practice to enjoy each and every moment is to pay attention to small pleasures. You can do this by creating enjoyable daily rituals like sitting with a cup of coffee in your garden every morning, taking a relaxing stroll in your neighborhood on Sundays, or making time to cuddle with your pets when you get home from work. You can also savor small pleasures by reducing multitasking, instead focusing all of your attention on one task at a time. For instance, while eating meals, put your phone on silent, switch off the TV, and enjoy each mouthful of your delicious meal.

Strategy 4: Focus on giving back to others and living a meaningful life.

Stress and anxiety have a way of making us feel isolated in the world and like we are the only people suffering. While comparing suffering is ludicrous, I do find that taking a moment to step out of my shoes and place myself in another person's makes me more grateful for the life I have (including the challenges that come with it). Giving back is the selfless act of putting another person's needs above your own. For a moment, their crisis is a matter of urgency and you do all that you can to assist in alleviating their suffering.

Not only is giving back emotionally fulfilling, but it also allows you to attract help from those who are more experienced, resourced, or knowledgeable than you for your own personal challenges. Thus, what you give freely to others you get back in ways that will astound you. You can give back by practicing random acts of kindness, volunteering, or using your strengths, skills, and talents to mentor someone else who could benefit from them.

Drop the Belittling Phrases

Part of reclaiming your power and putting an end to the onslaught of fear in your life is to pay careful attention to the words that you say. Since most of your interactions with others are based on verbal and non-verbal cues that have been a part of your programming for many years, it is possible to be in a less fearful place in your life but convey verbal messages that are belittling to who you are now. It's the same as losing a significant amount of weight but still carrying the same insecurities that you had when you were much heavier. It takes time for every part of your mind and body to come to the party, so this journey requires a lot of patience.

Below are some of the phrases that you may say automatically which convey a negative message about yourself, and also included are some ways to turn the situation around to be in your favor:

"I'm sorry."

Are you the type of person who apologizes when encountering awkward moments with people? Perhaps you bump into someone while shopping or take a few seconds longer to get into the elevator. This incessant need to apologize may be caused by a negative belief that another person's discomfort is your fault or your responsibility. This can also point to low self-esteem, regarding yourself as less important or valuable than others. You can control this need to apologize constantly by assessing whether the situation truly deserved an apology. Was what you did your fault or was it just a coincidence or natural error?

"It's just a case of luck."

Perhaps you are a person who responds to praise about your obvious achievements and successes with, "It's just luck." You may be doing this because you want to avoid coming off as arrogant or high-minded. However, watering down your achievements can be seen as dishonesty and a fake sense of modesty. The truth is that you worked very hard to achieve whatever goal it was and getting to this position took many years of rising and falling. A more confident statement would be one where you admit that you are successful, talented, or intelligent and simply end it with a "thank you". You deserve your moment to shine because you have earned the spotlight.

"I just…"

Some people are so good at defending themselves, even when it is inappropriate to do so. They can interpret someone else's opinion or compliment as a form of reproach or criticism. This makes them want to defend themselves or discredit what the other person was saying by responding with a statement starting with "I just…", or, "It's just…". For instance, they may respond to a compliment such as, "You look absolutely stunning!" with, "It's just a dress I borrowed from my sister." Instead of immediately discrediting what was said, take in the compliment or viewpoint, and respond with gratitude or another question seeking to understand the other person's views better.

"Probably/maybe/most likely/I'm not too sure."

Using words like "kind of", "maybe", or "I'm not too sure" is a way of sheltering yourself from possible backlash or disappointment if your views are seen as wrong. This may be brought about by the fear of failure, fear of rejection, or trying as much as possible to save yourself from public humiliation. Remember that no one's opinion is 100% true because we all see life through our own belief systems and life experiences. Therefore, when you are interested in something, especially when the topic is a passion of yours, feel free to speak in clear terms and claim your position on the matter. This will earn you people's respect for having such resolute opinions on certain subjects.

Four Fear-Busting Phrases to Repeat to Yourself Often

It is very difficult to think highly of yourself when you are burdened with so many worries and doubts in your life. And, generally, the less you engage in positive thinking, the more you start to witness your self-esteem dwindling. This type of scenario creates the perfect breeding ground for self-defeating beliefs to pop up and seize as much territory as they possibly can in your mind. However, it is also very difficult to maintain a positive view of yourself and your life without becoming consumed by your ego.

Perhaps the best solution to maintaining a positive outlook on your life without becoming egotistical is to practice mental habits that remind you of your own self-worth, forgetting about how others perceive you or what your contributions mean to others.

The following are four fear-busting and confidence-boosting phrases that will help you maintain high self-esteem.

"I am not the things I have/don't have."

In the global capitalist society that we live in, it is so easy for us to build our identities around objects. Of course, there is nothing wrong or bad with having possessions; however, it is important to distinguish yourself from what you have and don't have. For instance, if you have a prestigious job, remind yourself often that you are more than a job title, good salary, and validation from your peers. This recognition will free you from people-pleasing, compromising your values, or treating your career like it is all that you were born to do. On the other hand, if you are single and hope to find a partner and get married, remind yourself often that you are not defined by a romantic relationship. This recognition will free you from the desperation of finding a partner as it may cause you to lower your standards or allow unacceptable behavior from your partner.

"I am grateful for what I have."

When everything is going well in your life, it is easy to forget who you are and how far you have come. It's important to constantly remind yourself of the road you traveled to get to where you are today, because this mental playback will give you so much to be grateful for, as well as to keep you humble. Instead of just thinking about how grateful you are for what you have, you can go a step further and express your gratitude in a number of ways. For instance, you can write a gratitude letter, mentor someone much younger than you who could benefit from your learned wisdom, and regularly tell those closest to you how much you appreciate them.

"I don't put up with mistreatment from others."

One of the signs that you are a highly confident person is when you genuinely value yourself. This means that you don't allow other people to bring you down emotionally with their behaviors or actions. Every once in a while, take careful stock of your relationships and assess the quality of your interactions. Ask yourself what value you are receiving from being in certain relationships with those around you. Are you learning something new about yourself when you are with them? Do they make you feel comfortable to be yourself and share your thoughts and feelings freely? Do they offer supportive words and advice when it is necessary? It is not worth investing in relationships that are not reciprocal and feel one-sided.

After assessing your relationships, actively seek to spend more time with those people who bring value to your life (and vice versa), and distance yourself from those who are not as invested in learning about you and supporting you on your life's journey.

"I am aware of my response to certain stressful situations."

What is happening around you matters less than how you respond to what is happening around you. What you think about the stressful situations that occur in your life matters because it is the deciding factor determining how well you will cope with and overcome these challenges.

A really good habit to practice is reminding yourself often that you are the only one who can control your reactions. This means that instead of blaming the situation for unleashing your temper, you realize that unleashing your temper was a conscious or subconscious choice that you made as a way to deal with the stress. Understanding this will empower you to choose different ways to respond to stress—ones that are less destructive and that help you reach a productive outcome.

Practical Exercises to Release Fear

Being in a state of constant fear can feel like a death sentence. Some people have lived under its shadow for so long that they have forgotten what it feels like to be carefree and happy in each moment. No one deserves to be terrorized by fear or settle for a cautious life. You can experience a breakthrough from this feeling by practicing exercises that will help to put your mind at peace and feel more connected to your life.

Below are just a few exercises and techniques that will help you get rid of your fears as they arise throughout the day.

Believing for the Best: What If?

Fear comes as a result of us trusting in our own knowledge, skills, and strengths to pull us out of difficult situations. The moment we let go of trying to figure out a solution or manipulate the situation, there is an instant peace that washes over us.

Think about a recent situation that has been weighing you down emotionally and causing you to live in a perpetual state of fear. It may be a situation related to your finances, relationships, career, or medical condition. Think about the strong emotions you have been feeling, the quality of your thoughts, and the actions (or lack thereof) that you have taken.

With all this in mind, consider the following question: What would change if you knew that everything was going to work out in your favor, and in the end you would be laughing about this situation? How would this change how you feel, the thoughts flowing through your mind, and the actions that you would take? I assume that worrying would seem like a waste of your valuable time.

Relying on the mind to solve your problems or come up with a solution for something that is out of your control will cause panic and fear. This is because the mind hasn't been to the future yet and so it cannot conceive of what will happen next or how the outcome will turn out. Instead, it goes around in circles trying to find the best solutions from its archive of information but never really coming up with a conclusion. Asking yourself if everything will turn out well is a powerful way of canceling the numerous anxiety-producing "what if" questions that seek to terrify you about something that hasn't happened yet.

What if this is the situation that causes you to have a change of heart about your work? What if this is the person who has been sent to teach you a valuable lesson about life? What if this is the positive turning point for your health? What if this is the motivation you needed to prioritize your own self-development? What if there is something to learn from this pain?

Believing that everything is going to work out for your own good is the kind of thought that creates a mental shift, causing you to let go of wanting to control the situation and simply resting your mind. Imagine that there is a higher power who is at work 24/7 to turn good and bad situations that occur in your life into situations that are in your favor. If this higher power is doing so for you, it means that even when you are faced with a stressful situation, you can find an inner sense of peace and know that you will overcome it.

For this next part of the exercise, you will need a pen and paper to answer a few questions that you can also refer to when you are presented with a fearful situation. Give yourself enough time to answer the following questions:

1. Describe the situation that is bothering you right now. What kinds of fears are rising within you? What are the things that you have been thinking, feeling, and doing as a result of these fears?

2. How do you hope to feel once this situation has been taken care of?

3. How would you feel if you knew that everything was going to work out to your advantage? What kinds of thoughts would rush into your mind? What actions and plans would you make? What would you say to yourself?

Whenever you feel threatened by this type of situation again, refer to question number 3 and focus your mind on the feelings you would have if everything worked out well in the end. If you would like, you can also create positive affirmations to recite to yourself throughout the day and remind yourself of the beneficial outcomes that will follow this stressful or fearful situation.

Fear Processing Meditation

Meditation is an effective technique to process strong emotions and reduce the power they have over your mind. As you focus on the fear, for example, and allow it to be present within you, it stops becoming an unexplainable feeling of dread. Your fears are not as mean and ugly as you perceive them to be; all they want is to be shown love and then they will leave you in peace.

You can prepare for this guided meditation by sitting by yourself in a quiet room or out in a garden, removing anything that could become a distraction for you. Sit on the floor or on a chair with your back straight and arms resting on your lap. Gently close your eyes, and focus on slowing down your breathing. Take slow and deep breaths from your abdomen, inhaling for 4 counts, pausing for 4 counts, and exhaling for 4 counts. Repeat this counting process until you are completely relaxed. Start scanning your body from head to toe to locate the area where your fear is hiding. Assess each body part one at a time, and take a few minutes to thoroughly detect if any fear may be present there.

Once you find fear in your body, simply look at it without analyzing why it is there or whether it is appropriate for it to be present. As you look at your fear, allow it to feel welcome in your body, allowed to exist. If you sense the fear growing, allow it to do so. Also, notice what the fear feels like; it can have a physical sensation like a knot, pain, or tightness. It may also carry an emotional reaction like anxiety, sadness, or feeling out of control. If you find tears flowing down your face, allow them to flow without judging its appropriateness. Continue looking and feeling, completely open to your fear.

When you are ready, you can begin speaking to your fear in a warm, accepting, and compassionate voice:

Fear, you are welcome here. You are welcome here. You are welcome here.

Allow the fear to become whatever it does and simply look at it. If it desires to grow stronger and bigger, allow it to do this. Let the fear express itself to you in whatever form it decides to. It may recall words, memories, or thoughts from the past. Allow those thoughts to come to mind, and simply look at them without attaching yourself to them. If the fear moves locations in your body or decides to morph into another emotion, follow it, and welcome the new thoughts or emotions:

Thought/emotion, you are welcome here. You are welcome here. You are welcome here.

Now, allow yourself to come closer to the fear so that you can embrace it in whatever expression it has chosen. Give it gifts of love, understanding, compassion, and encouragement. Thank it for the positive aspects it has contributed to your life. When you are ready, you can release the fear from your body through meaningful breathing. As you breathe in, fill your lungs with the power of healing, and when you breathe out, focus your breath on the area where the fear is present. Do this until you the physical and emotional manifestations of fear vanish and you start feeling an emptiness where there was once that feeling.

The second part involves filling this empty space with love, peace, acceptance, and any other emotion you desire to take the place of fear. As you breathe in, fill your lungs with one positive emotion, and when you breathe out, focus your breath on the area where fear used to be. Do this for each emotion until you feel a fullness of love where fear was once present. Scan your body once again to assess if there are other places where fear may be hiding. If you find any, repeat the exercise again and release the fear. Repeat this exercise every day until you are no longer living each day in a fearful state.

Visualization Techniques

Anxiety can present itself in many forms, arriving without any notice and completely crippling your progress. Sometimes, it isn't so obvious, preferring to subtly invade your mind and nervous system, negatively affecting your ability to focus or adopt a positive mindset. One of the many powerful relaxation strategies is visualization. Visualization techniques help you manage stress and anxiety when they creep up on you suddenly. They activate the same neural networks that task performance does, thereby strengthening the connection between your mind and body.

The following are a few visualization techniques to try the next time you are feeling anxious.

1. The Relaxing Beach Scene Technique

Visualize yourself perched on a quiet sandy beach, seeing nothing but blue skies and gentle waves flowing back and forth. Take in the smell of the sea salt, the cool breeze hitting your face, and the sound of waves gathering. Imagine that your body is sinking deeper and deeper into the chair, becoming more at peace. Let go of any tension in your body, gently close your eyes, and breathe with the rhythm of the soothing waves.

2. The Blue Light Technique

Visualize your body insulated by a glowing blue light. Breathe in this light, and send it to your head, allowing it to completely illuminate your mind. Feel the transfer of love sent to your thoughts, beliefs, and ideas. As you breathe out, visualize tension from your mind leaving through your nostrils like black smoke. Continue to breathe in the blue light and send it to other areas of your body where you feel tension or anxiety such as your chest or heart area. Feel the transfer of love flowing to these other locations, and release tension through your nostrils.

3. Ball of Yarn Technique

Visualize a small ball of yarn holding all of the tension that you have accumulated throughout the day. Locate the tip of the yarn, and hold it as you gently push this ball away from you. Watch as the yarn begins to unravel and the tension within you becomes more and more insignificant. Continue to imagine that the yarn is unraveling until you feel completely calm and free of tension. When you are relaxed, imagine that the yarn has come to its end, resembling one long straight line.

4. The Liquid Quiet Technique

Visualize the word "quiet" as being a clear thick liquid that is gradually filling your head with peace and silence. See it pouring gently down your body until you feel totally immersed in gel-like liquid. Once your body is covered with peace and quiet, start practicing a breathing exercise or a guided meditation. Stay in this zone for as long as you need to.

5. Closing the Window Technique

Visualize a crowd of people talking loudly outside of your window. Perhaps what they are saying is inaudible or maybe they are hurling criticism, reminding you about past painful situations or pressuring you about other commitments. Instead of yelling at them or responding with your own insults, imagine yourself closing the window in a calm way (you may even draw the curtains if seeing the images of these people is triggering you in some way). Imagine that as soon as the window is tightly shut, the room becomes silent and the loud voices cease to exist. You can now enjoy your space without any mental distractions.

Chapter 7:

Mind-Body Strategies to Enhance Your Mental Focus

It can be difficult for adults with ADHD to maintain a consistent focus, especially when they are surrounded by various distractions. In today's digitally-connected world, distractions are just a click or swipe away. Even during moments of quiet time, distractions are close by, causing you to worry about tasks, plans, and outcomes that haven't even occurred yet. The ability to concentrate on a particular thing in your environment and direct all of your focus on it makes performing tasks easier.

I believe that it is possible for you to improve your mental focus by implementing mind-body strategies. However, this isn't an easy road to take. It requires you to commit to making mental and emotional adjustments to the way you think, process emotions, behave, and perceive yourself and your life.

Developing mental focus is not something that will happen after you finish reading this book or following a few months of consistent practice. Even the world's champion athletes have to continue to invest countless hours and practice in strengthening their concentration skills. Therefore, you can view your brain as a muscle that is currently flat and needs time and effort invested into it to pump it up and give it definition. We know that during normal physical training, muscle only appears after one has lost some fat. Similarly, your brain will become sharper after months of mind strengthening exercises that will soon become a habit.

In other words, you first need to dedicate yourself to the process of improving your mental focus before you can see any noticeable results. If you are still determined to travel on this natural mind-body healing journey, then you can start by penciling down a few healthy habits that you can incorporate into your daily life. Read some examples of habits below.

Habit 1: Focus on one task at a time.

While society celebrates multitasking, it can actually be an impediment when it comes to maintaining focus. When your brain is juggling many small individual tasks, it is easy for some of them to go unnoticed. Anyone who claims that they are good at multitasking is probably not placing their full attention on each task, which could lead to poor execution or a lot of errors during implementation. Decide that from now on, you will focus on one task at a time and regard it as the most important one in that moment until it is completed.

When distractions come to steal your attention, remind yourself that they are not as important as honing in your attention on this task. Think of your focus as being a spotlight. When you shine a spotlight in one area, everything else around it becomes dark and unnoticeable. The spotlight also allows you to see whatever is in the light very clearly. Thus, by focusing on single tasks at a time, you are able to be more productive and complete each one to the best of your ability.

Habit 2: Set your intentions for each day.

It is extremely helpful to give yourself something to focus on each day. This allows you to have a source of motivation for finishing tasks and facing challenges presented throughout the day. Setting intentions will help you decide early in the morning what kind of day you wish to have. These intentions will help boost your confidence and ground you when distractions become too consuming.

Giving yourself positive intentions to think about will also prevent your mind from spinning or being pulled in multiple directions. For instance, whenever you experience a stressful situation, you can bring to mind the intentions you set for that day to help you return to a state of clarity and calm.

Here are some powerful intentions that you can set for yourself:

- I will stay positive, even when I am challenged by new circumstances.
- I desire to get to know my colleagues better.
- I am open to learning something new.
- Maintaining steady breathing throughout the day is important to me.
- I will take a few deep breaths before I respond to another person.
- I want to smile more than I frown.
- I will be more open and honest in my communication.
- I intend on showing others the kind of acceptance I would like to be shown in return.
- I won't let fear stop me from continuing with my plans.
- I will do the best that I can today.

Habit 3: Incorporate more movement/exercise into your lifestyle.

Movement and exercise aren't only effective in keeping your body healthy, but they are also powerful strategies to help you clear your mind. Exercise has been known to reduce muscle tension, decrease stress, and boost your overall strength, self-confidence, and positive mentality (caused by the release of endorphins during exercise).

It is easier to commit to an exercise that you enjoy doing and that fits into your already established schedule. Avoid participating in activities that you perceive as a form of punishment or that make you dread performing the exercise. In essence, you are more likely to turn an activity that you love into a habit.

Habit 4: Create a nighttime ritual.

The best way to ensure that you have quality deep sleep is to make sure your body is well-rested and relaxed before bedtime. Thankfully, creating a nighttime routine that encourages this can help you sleep better in the long run. Everybody has their own method of winding down or activities that help them relax. This means that each person's nighttime routine will look different, and this is perfectly normal.

Here are a few suggestions of activities that you can incorporate into your custom nighttime ritual:

- Take a salt bath or have a shower meditation where you wash off the negative energy that may have attached itself to you throughout the day.

- Take time to spoil your body with aromatic body butters, a relaxing foot massage, or by dressing in your favorite pajamas.
- Find a quiet place to drink your decaffeinated tea and reflect on the day's activities.
- Catch up on some reading.
- Take time to write in your journal about what you experienced during your day.

Habit 5: Prioritize your calmness in all circumstances.

There are many triggers that you may be faced with throughout the day that could compromise your state of peace. It is important for you to prioritize your peace above any other factor or stressor. By maintaining your peace, you will be able to problem-solve more effectively, adopt a positive outlook on the situation, let go of trying to be in control of the outcome, and find an opportunity to express gratitude amidst a crisis.

There are many ways for you to guard your calmness as you go on about your daily activities, including the following:

- Avoid postponing your to-do list too long. If you are overwhelmed by the tasks, start by performing the easiest ones as this will give you the necessary motivation to tackle the more complex ones as you go. Stop being a starter, and start being a finisher.

- Learn how to say no more often, and schedule time every day for self-care and moments of silent reflection.
- Avoid being on your phone after a certain time at night (for example, 9:00 pm) in order to relax and prevent possible triggering information that will put your mind into overdrive.
- Find better alternatives to drinking coffee, and lower your intake of caffeine. Eating a well-balanced diet broken down into a number of meals and snacks throughout the day will provide you with more than enough natural energy to carry you through.

Mind-Body Exercises for Mental Focus

Mind-body exercises incorporate bodily movements, mental focus, and regulated breathing to improve a person's strength, balance, and overall well-being. There are five characteristics of mind-body exercises that set them apart from regular exercise; they are as follows:

- Concentrating on muscular movements
- Establishing an inner mental focus
- Synchronizing mind and body activity with breathing patterns

- The belief in life energy (also known as chi, source, or a higher power)
- Bringing attention to form and alignment

Any mind-body exercise you perform will include one or more of the characteristics mentioned above. Thus, the greatest difference between mind-body exercises and regular physical exercise is the intentionality behind each movement. With physical exercise, your intention may be to maintain good health or lose weight, but with mind-body exercises, your intention is always to restore or create a sense of peace between your mind and your body. Peace between these two entities helps you live a more fulfilling and emotionally stable life, which also promotes good mental, emotional, and physical health. Below are a few mind-body exercises that you can try out and incorporate into your lifestyle.

Relaxation Techniques: The Body Scan

Relaxation techniques are a great way to naturally improve mental focus and reduce stress. Relaxation isn't purely about being calm or enjoying a particular hobby. It is also a respected practice for treating the effects of stress on your mind and body.

Typically, relaxation techniques involve redirecting your attention to something soothing and bringing more awareness to your body. A body scan is a type of relaxation technique that blends both controlled breathing with progressive muscle regulation. After a few minutes of slow and deep breathing, you focus your awareness on various parts of your body at a time. As you focus on specific parts, you mentally release any physical or emotional pain that may be stored in those areas. Here is an example of a typical body scan that you can follow at home:

Begin by bringing your attention to your body. Gently close your eyes, and notice how your body feels seated on the floor or a chair. Notice any tension or resistance in your body. Now take a few deep breaths, and as you inhale each breath, imagine new life is entering your body. As you exhale, allow all of the physical and emotional tension to be emptied out of you. Notice your feet making contact with the floor, the weight of your arms, and how your back feels against a chair.

Bring your focus to your stomach area, and assess whether there is discomfort there. Soften this area by inhaling life energy and directing this energy toward your stomach area. Imagine that new life is being established in your stomach region. Notice your hands and fingers, and assess if there is any tension there. Feel the sensations in your arms—their heaviness and how effortlessly they are hanging. Scan for other areas of your body where you may have tension. If you notice tightness in your neck and throat region, for instance, simply inhale life energy. As you exhale, direct this energy toward your neck and throat area.

Imagine that the tension is diffused by this pure healing energy and that in its place you have new life. Once you have completely scanned your entire body, notice the full presence of your body. Take one more deep breath in and out, and gently open your eyes.

Guided Imagery: Visualizing Increased Focus and Memory Recollection

Research has shown that guided imagery is an effective technique to use for decreasing anxiety, lowering pain, and helping to bring about a sense of mental clarity, strength, and control. It involves using your imagination to create scenes or experiences in your mind that can help with stress management and improving focus. If you are doing it on your own, choose to imagine scenes or experiences that carry significance for you and can make you feel instantly calm.

For example, you can think back to a moment that made you feel good about yourself or where you successfully accomplished a task through sustained focus. Alternatively, you can imagine a fictitious experience where you have optimum focus and find it easy to concentrate on, plan, and strategize your goals.

At its core, guided imagery is all about reinforcing a positive vision of yourself where you are performing or living as your ideal self. For those who find it difficult to conjure up mental images, you can rely on guided imagery scripts that can be accessed online. Below is a script guiding you through the process of writing an exam that will help you visualize yourself as having clear focus and high levels of concentration and being productive.

Sit in a comfortable position on the floor or on a chair, and allow your body to completely relax. You may notice a few distractions in your environment that are causing you to fidget around. Gently move your focus away from them by focusing on your breathing. First, start by noticing the rhythm of your breathing— whether it is fast, irregular, or slow. Take a few deep breaths in and let them out, noticing the rhythm of your breathing becoming slower and more consistent.

If you notice tension in your body, gently focus your breathing where it lies, and using deep and slow breaths, release the tension completely. When you are finally feeling calm and your entire body feels relaxed and heavy, begin to visualize the process of preparing to write an exam. Imagine yourself feeling motivated to write this exam because you have thoroughly studied the subject. See yourself as an expert on the subject, and feel the enthusiasm rushing into you as you prepare to share the wealth of wisdom you have gathered on this subject.

If this image makes you want to smile or laugh, feel free to show these expressions openly. Now, begin to visualize the preparation process you undertook to write this exam. Imagine yourself sitting in your favorite place, having your favorite study snacks, and feeling encouraged to learn. Picture your mind being open to absorbing as much information as possible. See it effortlessly absorbing information and retaining it like a sponge. See yourself smiling or celebrating the relationship you have with your mind. Picture the intimate conversations you have with it leading up to moments like this. Imagine saying this to your mind: "You are my friend. I appreciate everything you do for me."

Now, imagine that you are finally studying. Instead of information being transferred to your mind through your eyes, imagine that it is transferred through each breath you take. Each time you take a deep breath in, information is sent effortlessly to your brain and stored in a safe place labeled "study notes", and with every exhale, you are letting go of any anxiety or stress related to the studying process.

Picture yourself enjoying the process of learning new information. You are confident and highly capable. See yourself engaging with the study material and remembering every word, phrase, and sentence with ease. See yourself studying several times and feeling energized the more time you spend with your books. Imagine yourself reading the material, listening to it, and publicly sharing it with others who are just as passionate about the subject as you are. Now, imagine that it is the day of the exam. You are feeling highly driven and grateful for the experience to share everything that you have learned and successfully retained.

Try to imagine the amount of peace you have while opening the test paper and seeing everything that you studied presented to you. Every answer that you write is written with clarity and consideration. You can easily draw upon the information and even give fresh insight when required. Imagine yourself having that "aha" moment at the end of the exam that you have done exceedingly well on. You are certain that you have done a great job; you just *know* it.

Now that you have finished taking the exam, you are feeling so proud of yourself. Imagine telling yourself that you are proud of yourself. You are feeling calm and confident while you wait for your test to come back.

Next, imagine that you have just received your exam results. Feel the excitement as you prepare to see how well you've done. Picture seeing "congratulations!" in bold print. You have passed with flying colors. You've received a better grade than you had anticipated. This is above and beyond your expectations. Well done! You did a stellar job. Enjoy this feeling of accomplishment and success. Take a few deep breaths, and truly bask in this moment. Imagine yourself being determined to take another exam just to experience this feeling again.

When you are ready, you can gently open your eyes and begin waking up the rest of your body. You can continue to sit in this position and reflect on your experience until you are ready to get up and continue with the rest of your day.

Focused Meditation: Concentration on Breath

Focused meditation can improve your levels of concentration by training you to focus on an object, sound, or bodily sensation instead of trying to get you to clear your mind. Focusing on something intently allows you to stay in the present moment and naturally reduce or eliminate the constant internal dialogue or flow of thoughts. Unlike classic meditation where the objective is to gently quiet your mind, focused meditation urges you to direct your attention to one thing completely. It takes only five steps to successfully carry out a focused meditation. These five steps may be new to you now; however, over time, it will be easier to recall and practice them.

Begin practicing your focused meditations for five minutes at a time and gradually work your way up as you become better at holding your focus for longer periods of time. You can carry out these short sessions anywhere and at any time of the day, provided that they are administered in a quiet place with little to no distractions around. Below is a short focused meditation that will ask you to direct all of your attention to your breath.

Get yourself in a comfortable position. Ensure that you are sitting upright, sinking your body into a chair, or on the floor. Notice the natural heaviness of your body and tension being released as you start to relax more and more. Loosen your shoulders and begin taking deep and meaningful breaths from your belly.

Instead of thinking about your breathing, experience it. Enjoy how it begins and the physiological change that takes place in your body as your lungs expand. Notice how relaxing every exhale is and how your body becomes even calmer. Notice the air coming in and out of your nostrils and the pace at which air is inhaled and exhaled. Pay attention to the full cycle of breathing and every natural pause in between.

If you find that your internal voice is creating a story around this meditation, analyzing your breath, or bringing up other stressful situations of the day, gently shift your attention back to your breathing, and enjoy the free sensations that you experience from this soothing exercise. If you get distracted again, gently shift your attention back to your breathing; do this as many times as needed. Keep your mind focused on your breathing until the five-minute period is complete. To end the focused meditation, take three slightly longer and deeper breaths, and then open your eyes when you are ready.

Art Therapy for Improving Concentration

Art therapy is an effective and fun therapy to use for taming impulsivity, distractibility, and anxiety. It uses creative processes like drawing, painting, building a craft, or sculpting to improve focus and levels of confidence in those living with ADHD. Art therapy is based on the assertion that self-expression through creativity is an effective way of addressing emotional pain, improving interpersonal skills, reducing stress, and increasing self-awareness. Art therapy is recommended for both old and young people, and it doesn't require you to be the next Picasso. The emphasis is on exploring emotional problems through a creative activity and sensory integration.

During the creative process, various parts of your brain will be engaged. For instance, sweeping a paintbrush across a blank piece of paper requires motor skills, and drawing a picture of a past memory or emotion requires you to use analytical and sequential operations and reasoning. Moreover, throughout the process of creating art, you will be fully engaged in the task, over time improving your attention skills and working memory.

The process of making art is also useful for stress management because as you draw, paint, or sculpt, you become more relaxed. It is also a known fact that creative expression increases your levels of serotonin (the hormone governing your moods, feelings, and overall well-being) and reduces the risk of depression and anxiety. The key to achieving all of these health benefits through art therapy is to enjoy the process of making art instead of seeing it as a way to reach a final product. There is no need to make a perfect drawing because your art is about sharing how you feel. When you find yourself too caught up in the details while making art, take a few deep breaths, and connect with how the process of creating art is making you feel.

It is also important to be curious and avoid judging yourself on the work you are creating. If the artwork doesn't come out how you would have liked, focus on what you can do differently the next time you have an opportunity to creatively express yourself. If you are curious about what art therapy entails, you can try out some of the creative art projects listed below to help you improve your mind and body connection.

Creative Exercises to Deal With Emotion

- Draw or paint your emotions, focusing entirely on what you're feeling in the moment.
- Create an emotional wheel by using color and expressing each emotion vividly.
- Create a stress painting by painting a picture using colors that represent your stress, anger, or frustration.
- Put together an art journal where you document your daily experiences through elaborate drawings.
- Make use of line art. This is a basic form of creative expression, but it can allow you to convey a lot of emotion by demonstrating how you are feeling.
- Design a postcard that you never intend on sending. It can express the anger, disappointment, or rejection you feel from a painful situation.
- Draw a large heart on a page, and fill the heart with all of the emotions you are feeling right now.

Creative Exercises to Help You Relax

- Paint while listening to soothing music, and allow your body to fully relax.
- Make an elaborate scribble drawing using lines, colors, and your wild imagination.

- Get your hands messy, and have fun with finger painting.
- Draw a picture in the dark, and allow yourself to express the full range of emotion you are feeling without having the ability to judge your creation.
- Draw something on a very large scale and something else on a very small scale, requiring you to get your whole body involved. For instance, you can paint a large mural on a wall or paint a delicate clay teacup.
- Create your own vision board using picture cutouts, and arrange them in a collage.
- Color in a drawing template or one that allows you to color in numbers.

Creative Exercises to Help You Feel Happy

- Draw your idea of a perfect day, thinking about all of the things that constitute a perfect day for you.
- Take photographs of things, places, and people that you believe are beautiful and make you happy. No one else is required to like these photos besides you. You can print and frame your photography around your home, giving you a source of inspiration every day.
- Make a drawing that is the visual representation of your favorite quote.

- Create a painting, drawing, or sculpture representing what freedom means to you.

- Have you ever had a spiritual experience? Illustrate it using color, texture, and powerful keywords.

- Sew a stuffed animal that you can cuddle with when you are feeling low. Pick an animal that's symbolic to you in some way and that will make you feel happy and at peace when you see it.

- Creatively document a time when you did something that you didn't think you were capable of doing. Use this experience to celebrate an act or moment of extreme courage in your life.

Creative Exercises for Improving Self-Awareness

- Draw images of every good trait you have that you can think of.

- Draw yourself as an animal. Choose one that you believe represents who you are or what you stand for.

- On a large piece of paper, draw a timeline and insert photos (you can draw them if you don't have physical copies) of the most significant moments in your life.

- Make a sculpture of your ideal self. It doesn't necessarily have to be based on your body; it can be inspired by your ideal state of mind or your emotional identity.

- Paint the different aspects of your personality, moods, and beliefs.
- Make art using your unique fingerprint. Take ink and a blank canvas, and make an image using only your inked fingers.
- Draw yourself as a tree, placing keywords that form the basis of who you are at the roots, your good qualities as the trunk, and aspects of yourself that you are trying to change as the leaves.
- Paint a childhood memory that holds significance for you. In your painting, highlight what was so important or powerful about this memory. If you have unresolved emotions about it, add those as well, showing how they connect to the whole situation.

Creative Exercises to Express Gratitude

- If you cannot put your gratitude in words, document it visually. Create a collage of what you are most grateful for today, within the last six months, or throughout the course of your life.
- Create a family tree, honoring the friends and family members who have been your greatest sources of support and strength.
- Make a piece of art or a sculpture for someone else to show them how much you appreciate them.

- Write down each letter of a person's name, and find words that start with the same letter of the alphabet that symbolize what they mean to you. You can send them the list on a special occasion or as one of your random acts of kindness.

Conclusion

There is so much research available on the internet about mental health conditions, including what they are, how they are caused, and how to treat the symptoms that may arise. When I was writing this book, I was not short on articles and research informing me about ADHD and the devastating impact it can have on an individual's life. However, the information that I have put together in this book was very difficult to find.

This is because the intention of *The Science of Destroying Adult ADHD* wasn't written to predict a gloomy future ahead for you or to remind you of all of the experiences that you have missed out on as a result of your mental condition; the sole emphasis of this book was to offer you hope and convince you through each chapter that it is possible for you to lead a fulfilling life with or without your diagnosis. I find it strange that there are only a handful of books that are bold enough to make this claim and dispel the myth that living with a mental health condition signifies the beginning of the end.

I am certain that you have found this book refreshing with the twist it has taken on speaking about adult ADHD. However, if there are a few things that you should remember from this book, they are as follows:

1. **There Is Nothing Wrong With You**

You are no less of a human because you live with ADHD, nor does your mental health condition mean that you need to settle for a subpar life. There is truly nothing wrong with you. Your condition is not shameful, immoral, or embarrassing. You deserve as much respect and exposure to the same opportunities that anyone else would receive. For many years, you may have lived with feelings of guilt or a low sense of self-worth because you believed in the social stigmas and judgments that were made about people living with your condition. Now, being more knowledgeable about who you are, you have yet another chance to choose what you will think about yourself and your condition. Choose beliefs that empower you to aim higher and set even bigger goals.

2. Your Body Knows How to Heal Itself

With you every day of your life is a self-healing machine that's also known as your body. Throughout the ages, the human body has constantly evolved to adapt to new environments and protect itself from new threats. Your body is still evolving and learning new ways of correcting old programmings, self-defeating beliefs, and behaviors that have been harmful to your well-being. I don't believe that your body needs any help from synthetic drugs to successfully heal itself from past infirmities. However, it does need your willingness to allow it to heal. Giving your body the space and time to heal means being open to listening when your body shares messages about how it is feeling. For so long, you might have ignored these natural signals or believed they were insignificant. These messages are clues about what your body needs to improve its health and function at its optimum ability. Listen to your body, and let it do all of the work.

3. **Self-Awareness Is the Beginning of a Life Not Governed by Your Condition**

If self-awareness was medicine, I would prescribe you high doses of it because it is the most powerful human trait to have. Being self-aware allows you to see yourself outside of what you are feeling and thinking. You begin to realize that you are not your thoughts and feelings but rather the one who stands observing their thoughts and feelings. Self-awareness is your gateway to a life free from fear, stress, anxiety, and low self-esteem, because once you recognize the patterns of negative thinking, you are able to rectify the thoughts and emotions that you have about yourself and your life. You are no longer hopeless, living as a victim of ADHD symptoms. Building self-awareness will give you power over your moods, thoughts, and actions and cause you to choose the quality of your life experiences.

I hope that you take all that you have learned from this book and see it as the starting point of a life-long journey seeking mental and emotional freedom. You can refer back to it whenever you need a firm reminder that you are valuable just as you are. Feel free to share this book with friends and family members who may be living with ADHD or provide support for someone living with the condition.

Remember to always treat your healing as a work in progress, committing every day to hearing and reading positive and encouraging words similar to the ones you read in this book. Continue living life to the best of your ability and learning from every circumstance, whether it is bad or good. I know that you were built to survive all of the obstacles that life throws at you, but you need to believe this about yourself, too!

Thank you for reading This book.

If you enjoyed it please visit the site where you purchased it and write a brief review. Your feedback is important to me and will help other readers decide whether to read the book too.

Thank you!

Michelle Martin